ABC of The Keto Diet

The Only Ketogenic Diet Guide You'll Ever Need for Superfast Metabolism, Instantly Visible Fat Loss, and Permanent Low Carb Healthy Lifestyle Habits.

BEN CENA

© **Copyright 2022 - All rights reserved.**

The content inside this book may not be duplicated, reproduced, or transmitted without direct written permission from the author or publisher.

Under no circumstances will any blame or legal responsibility be held against the publisher, or author, for any damages, reparation, or monetary loss due to the information contained within this book, either directly or indirectly.

Legal Notice:

This book is copyright protected. It is only for personal use. You cannot amend, distribute, sell, use, quote or paraphrase any part, or the content within this book, without the consent of the author or publisher.

Disclaimer Notice:

Please note the information contained within this document is for educational and entertainment purposes only. All effort has been executed to present accurate, reliable, up to date, complete information. No warranties of any kind are declared or implied. Readers acknowledge that the author is not engaging in the rendering of legal, financial, medical, or professional advice. The content within this book has been derived from various sources. Please consult a licensed professional before attempting any techniques outlined in this book.

By reading this document, the reader agrees that under no circumstances is the author responsible for any losses, direct or indirect, that are incurred as a result of the use of the information contained within this document, including, but not limited to, errors, omissions, or inaccuracies.

TABLE OF CONTENT

CHAPTER 1: Introduction to the Keto Lifestyle 5

    What Is Keto? A Brief Explanation and History 8

    Why Would Keto Be the Best Option? 11

    Can the Ketogenic Diet Be Your Lifestyle? 14

CHAPTER 2: Starting Keto 18

    How to Start Keto 18

    Counting the Macros 21

    Counting Net Carbohydrates 23

    Too Much? 26

    Every Person Is Different 29

    Keto Macro Formula 33

    Type and Amount of Water 40

CHAPTER 3: Guide 44

    Keto at Home 46

    Keto Outside of the House 47

    How to Cheat 50

CHAPTER 4: The Pros and Cons of Keto 54

    The Cons of Keto 54

    The Pros of Keto 56

CHAPTER 5: Usual Mistakes 59

    What Are the Usual Mistakes People Make on Keto? 60

CHAPTER 6: Supplementation 66

Do You Need to Supplement Keto? 67

What Supplements Do You Need When You're Doing Keto?
..68

CHAPTER 7: Keto Compared to Other Diets 73

A Case for Keto Being the Best Diet Plan Out There 73

What Sets Keto Apart from Others? 74

CHAPTER 8: Beginner Keto Meal Plan 77

Sample Three-Day Meal Plan for an Overweight Male Adult
..78

Sample Three-Day Meal Plan for Average Athletic Female
Adult..86

SUMMARY 94

CONCLUSION 99

Want to Stop Carb Cravings Instantly and Effortlessly?

Scan This QR code with your smartphone or tablet and Get Your FREE GIFT NOW!

CHAPTER 1:
Introduction to the Keto Lifestyle

Unless you have been living under a rock in the last few years, it's very much likely that you have already heard of people going on the keto diet. And if you indulge in actually reading this book in its entirety, you will come to discover why the keto diet has grown to become so popular these days, especially for people who are looking to keep fit and trim. You will also find that the keto philosophy is going to be so much more than a general guideline for what kind of food you should be putting into your mouth. That's why this chapter is worded the way that it is.

"Going keto" is more than just adopting a dietary guideline for yourself. It's the adoption of a lifestyle. It truly is a revolutionary and structural principle that can dramatically alter a person's overall health and wellness for the better.

What a lot of people don't understand about health and wellness is that there are no Band-Aid solutions or quick fixes to any physical issues or conditions that you might have. There is no "secret sauce" or "magic bean" that can instantly yield positive results pertaining to your health and fitness. Being physically fit isn't just about making a conscious choice to eat a salad every once in a while. Choosing to be physically fit is a lifestyle choice that you have to own up to with your whole self. It's the sum of all the habits and choices that you make in your daily life.

You might find it corny, but being fit and healthy truly is a lifestyle. You will find out that so many people in this world are experiencing deteriorating standards and states of health purely because of the lifestyle choices that they make. Studies have shown that only 33% of kids have active lifestyles these days. Only around 5% of adults take part in the recommended thirty minutes of vigorous physical activity every day, and only a third of adults actually achieve the recommended amount of healthy physical activity within a week.

This might be very uncomfortable for a lot of people to hear, but technology has essentially rendered society to become more physically inactive. Studies have shown that kids who traditionally used to spend most of their time outside playing with other kids now spend most of their days in front of screens, like phones, televisions, and computers. This is the reason that more and more kids are bordering on becoming obese even at such early ages.

But it's not just the kids who are becoming victims to the technology that they use in their everyday lives. Adults rely a lot on cars and mass transport systems for their daily commutes. Fewer and fewer people are running, cycling, or even walking these days because of the abundance of various transportation options. Based on the data made available by the Office of National Statistics, a rising number of people these days are being diagnosed with "lifestyle cancers," meaning cancers that are acquired through lifestyle choices and habits.

To further illustrate the gravity of this point, a Canadian scientist has suggested that more people are actually essentially killing themselves with the choices that they make for themselves day in and day out. According to Dr. Doug Manuel, a professor at the University of Ottawa and a senior scientist at the Ottawa Hospital, unhealthy habits like smoking, drinking, and physical inactivity result in as much as half the deaths of Canadians annually. He also said that the practice of these habits could decrease life expectancy by as much as six years.

And in the face of all these statistics and numbers, it can feel rather discouraging and sad to know that so many people are decreasing the length and quality of their lives because of the choices that they make. But you shouldn't fret. There are also some very convincing numbers that show that there is a critical mass of individuals who are taking health and wellness very seriously. With enough guidance and commitment, it can be very easy to propagate and grow this critical mass of individuals into a global movement that can potentially change the world for the better.

You may consider this book to be a contribution to that movement of further improving the state of health and physical fitness in society today. As you further unfurl this book page by page, you will come to discover this entire piece's mission to drive people into adopting healthier lifestyles overall. And even though the primary mission is to make a case for the keto lifestyle to become a universal norm, the ultimate goal is to improve the overall health of the world that we live in, whether it's through keto principles or not.

The fact of the matter is that living a life of fun and fulfillment doesn't necessarily have to come at the expense of your health and fitness. This is a common misconception that a lot of people have when it comes to adopting healthier lifestyle habits. This is common advocacy that many proponents and practitioners of the keto diet would like to emphasize to nonbelievers and agnostics in the world of dieting and healthy living. Choosing to be healthy shouldn't be seen as a chore or as an inconvenience. In fact, the opposite should be true. Choosing to adopt healthy habits should be seen as a supplement to living a full and happy life.

Dealing with sickness, unhealthiness, and even potential death can be a very big hurdle to living a happy life. That is why choosing to have fun and deciding to be well should always go hand in hand with each other. One can't exist without the other. One must always be able to conflate being healthy with having fun because neither can be sustainable when just practiced on its own.

And that can essentially be the thesis for the keto lifestyle. It's a healthy practice that doesn't make you feel like you are being restricted, suffocated, or chained to boring and bland lifestyles in order for you to get healthier. Let this chapter be the start of the journey that we embark upon together—a journey toward a healthier and happier you through the keto lifestyle.

What Is Keto? A Brief Explanation and History

Okay, so it might be best for us to get the basics covered first. This section in the book is going to seek to orient you on what the basic fundamentals and principles are surrounding the keto diet. It's very important that before you actually adopt the keto diet for your own life, you are able to gain a deep and profound understanding of what it is and why it's an effective dietary plan. It can be very tempting to just pull up a diet plan from the Internet and follow it to a tee. But if you don't first prepare yourself by understanding the basics and principles behind the diet, then it's likely that you would either end up doing it wrong or not be able to sustain it for the long term.

Remember that in any aspect of life, you conduct yourself with structure and purpose. This is the only way that you would ever be able to ensure that your actions become habits and not just random practices that happen way too infrequently. With that, you would never be able to structure your life with keto diet principles unless you first understand what these principles are. This section of the book is going to highlight to the reader the need-to-know details of the keto diet and will help prepare you for the other concepts that are going to be covered in this book.

So let's answer this question: What exactly is the keto diet?

Well, to start with, the term "keto" is actually derived from the words "ketones" or "ketosis" in the body. In a nutshell, the keto diet is designed to induce a state of ketosis in the body.

Ketosis is a physical state in which there is an abundance of ketones through a human's bodily system. Ketones are very small molecules in the body that serve as an alternative source of energy for human beings to carry out physical activity. Ketones only ever really come into play whenever there is a shortage of glucose or sugar within the body that is needed to sustain prolonged bodily function.

The only way to induce a state of ketosis within the body is if one reduces their consumption of carbohydrates to an extremely minimal degree. This is because of the fact that carbs are so quickly broken down and converted into blood sugar, which the body needs to function properly. In order to achieve ketosis, it's also important to limit the consumption of protein to a moderate amount as excess protein can also be converted into blood sugar.

The liver is the primary culprit in the production of ketones in the human body. These ketones are then utilized to fuel the body whenever blood sugar levels are low. Even brain function is greatly dependent on fuel that comes from ketones when there is a shortage of glucose in the body. Take note that the brain is going to require a lot of energy in order for your body to function properly. Keep in mind that the brain is essentially the entire command center and operating system for your body. If your brain isn't working right, your entire body is going to feel off. And there are only two things that can power the brain: glucose and ketones.

When you strictly adhere to keto diet principles, your body is going to be caught in a perpetual state of ketosis, and whenever your body is in a state of ketosis, it's going to use up your ketones as a fuel source. This means that your body is going to heighten its burning of fat in order to compensate for the low glucose and insulin levels. Once you are in a state of ketosis, the storage of fat within your body becomes a lot more accessible, so it helps optimize the entire fat-burning process.

Naturally, from the information that has been covered, the keto diet is great for people who are looking to shed a little weight and burn off that extra fat. But there are also other health benefits that might not be so obvious right away. For one, being on a keto diet is going to stave off hunger pangs because the food you consume is going to satiate you and help you feel fuller for longer. And secondly, in a state of ketosis, you are given a steady flow of energy, which can help keep you alert, focused, and active.

Of course, there are other ways in which a person can reach a state of ketosis. A strict fast and abstinence from the consumption of food would be such an option. However, it's virtually impossible for anyone to fast forever without dying. That is why the keto diet continues to serve as the most effective and sustainable way to induce a state of ketosis within the body.

Even though the keto diet has seemingly only recently emerged in its popularity, it is actually a dietary concept that has been around for quite a while already at this point. The earliest recorded scientific study surrounding the keto diet was actually in 1921 in a project spearheaded by Dr. Russell Wilder from the Mayo Clinic.

There had been previous studies that suggested that patients who suffered from epilepsy actually benefited from engaging in fasting and starvation. There was a documented decrease in the rate of seizures and epileptic episodes whenever a patient engaged in a long fast. However, the fasting was never sustainable, and so scientists decided to try to venture into alternative methods of inducing the same effects without having patients lock into an indefinite fast.

In 1921, Dr. Russell decided to look into how the keto diet might actually affect patients who were suffering from epilepsy. He had already been using the same methodology to induce a state of ketosis in diabetic patients. By the year 1924, Dr. Peterman from the Mayo Clinic was already incorporating the keto diet into his treatments regularly for his patients. The keto diet then became a primary tool in battling epilepsy and seizure episodes in people. But as more effective and less costly anti-seizure medication was brought into the market, the popularity of the keto diet gradually decreased over time.

However, toward the start of the 1990s, there was a revived interest in the keto diet because of Dr. John Freeman at Johns Hopkins. In a study that he had conducted in 1992, he claimed that the diet actually induced a full seizure control in around 30% of children who had previously had uncontrolled seizures. One of the kids who had shown positive results in that study was Charles Abrahams. His thankful parents would later go on to found the Charlie Foundation, which spearheaded the popularization of the keto diet in contemporary times.

Why Would Keto Be the Best Option?

We always want to have the best things that life possibly has to offer. Whenever the newest iPhone is released, we always want to buy it because Apple's marketing tells us that it's the best iPhone out on the market. Whenever we buy tickets to a concert, we always aim for getting front-row seats because we are told that they're the best seats in the house. Whenever we're looking to buy a new car, we enter a car dealership and test-drive various makes and models to make sure that we can get the best car that we could possibly afford.

As human beings, it's normal for us to want the best thing that could possibly be made available to us. So when you're in search of a new health-and-fitness regimen, it's already expected that you would want the best possible one for you to adopt in your own life. You don't want to play games when it comes to your health after all. You're not up for trying anything that would be too risky or ineffective. You don't want to be compromising your health or your time for any health and fitness fads out there that won't really be generating a positive impact on your life.

Health and wellness is an investment that you choose to make in yourself. You are going to have to invest a lot of time, money, effort, commitment, and energy into making sure that you are as healthy as can be. That is why it always makes sense that you will always want to be yielding the best possible returns for your investment when it comes to the diet that you will adopt for yourself.

But is the keto diet out there the best possible option for you to have?

Well, yes and no.

Confusing? Let me explain.

It would be normal for you to be skeptical about the claim that the keto diet is the absolute best option out there for every single person.

It's always really hard to gauge the effectiveness of a diet in universal and general terms. That's why a lot of people in the scientific community will tend to avoid making sweeping statements like this when making a case for a particular scientific paradigm and theory. It would be arrogant to think that there is a single diet on this earth that would serve as the best diet for everyone who resides in it.

And the actual truth when it comes to dieting and fitness?

The best diet and fitness program in the world is the one that works best for you.

It's as simple as that.

Keto is definitely a popular diet nowadays because it has worked for so many people in the past. And undoubtedly, it's going to work for more and more people as we emerge into the future. However, we must not discount the number of people who have tried getting into the keto lifestyle and just failed to achieve the results that they wanted for themselves. This might not necessarily mean that the diet is ineffective and flawed beyond consideration.

There are just certain people whose lifestyles, preferences, outlooks, philosophies, or general practices just make it impossible for them to find success in the keto diet. This is not the fault of the person, nor is it the fault of the keto diet in general. Sometimes, it's just not a good fit.

There are plenty of other dietary programs and paradigms out there that are up for trying, and we're going to touch on some of them later on. But for now, you just have to keep in mind that just because one particular philosophy or methodology doesn't work for you doesn't mean that you're doomed to live a life of compromised physical health and wellness.

Different Strokes for Different Folks

Again, it's important to reiterate that we are all unique in our practices, goals, situations, means, resources, schedules, priorities, perspectives, and worldviews. That comes with the territory of being a normal human being. No two people are alike, and it would be downright foolish to assume that just because the keto diet works for one person, it's automatically going to work for everyone else. We are all going to respond to different methodologies in a number of different ways. It's just important that you actually adopt a fitness philosophy that works well for you and allows for you to see tangible results with regard to strengthening your overall physical condition.

There is no tangible or plausible scientific study, experiment, project, or data in the world that would be able to prove that the keto diet is one that is absolutely meant for everyone. There are just some of us who might be built for it, and there will be some of us who aren't. For some people, the keto diet might actually be the best thing to ever happen to them. For others, it might be the worst. Again, it's just going to be a different experience for every single person.

But that doesn't mean that the keto diet can't make a strong case for itself relative to other forms of dieting out there. As you make your way through this book, you are going to gain a better and deeper understanding of what the keto diet is and why it really is so effective to large sums of people. You're also going to come to discover why it's such a preferred vehicle for a lot of people on the road to optimal health and wellness. So yes, the keto diet may not be the best diet out there for every single person in the world, but it certainly brings a lot of things to the table. And it would be difficult to deny the fact that it is a powerful force in the health-and-wellness industry.

The only way you would ever be able to find out if the keto diet is actually the best diet in the world is if you try it out for yourself. And if you're interested in doing so, then this book is going to help guide you through the whole process so that you can be sure that you are doing things properly and that you are maximizing all the potential benefits of the diet itself. It all starts with you determining whether the keto diet would be a good fit for your lifestyle.

Can the Ketogenic Diet Be Your Lifestyle?

Again, it's all about being able to adopt the keto diet for your own lifestyle. And given the vast enormity of the world and the diversity of the people who reside in it, not everyone is going to have the same kind of positive reaction to keto principles. Does that mean that the keto diet is bad? No. It just isn't going to be the right match sometimes.

It's like going to the store and finding a really nice-looking shirt. You know that the shirt looks great, so you decide to try it on. But then once you look at yourself in the mirror, you see certain aspects of the shirt that don't look good on you. The sleeves are too short. The collar is too big. The color doesn't complement your skin color well. It just isn't a good fit. That doesn't mean that the shirt is bad or that it wouldn't look good on someone else. It just isn't the shirt for you. And it's exactly the same with how diets work. There are just some people who are better suited for certain diets than others.

This segment of the chapter is going to delve into whether the keto diet would be a good fit for your own lifestyle or not. Admittedly, as amazing and as powerful as the keto diet really is, it's just not something that would be suited for every single person in the world. So not to belabor the point any longer, let's get right down to it. Let us discover if you would be able to adopt the keto diet for your life or not.

Who Is It For?

Ultimately, for the most part, the keto diet is a dietary principle that is designed to induce a state of ketosis in a human being's body. Ketosis is the process in which the body turns to its stored fats and converts it into energy to fuel the body's daily functions. Therefore, with that in mind, a lot of people turn to the keto diet in order to achieve their weight loss goals.

So who is the primary target of the keto diet?

Mostly, obese or overweight people would do well with the keto diet. The general public is probably well aware by now of the dangers and risks that come with carrying extra fat in the body. Obesity is no joke, and it can lead to a lot of serious physical illnesses and conditions for people. Studies have already shown that people who are obese or overweight are more prone to the following health problems:

- diabetes
- high blood pressure
- cancer
- stroke
- kidney disease
- sleep apnea
- fatty liver disease
- osteoarthritis

When there is excess fat in the body, it can compromise the overall integrity of the human body. This is where the keto diet comes in. If paired with proper exercise and portion control, inducing a state of perpetual ketosis in the body can really aid in the fat-burning process. Instead of having to rely on the consumption of carbohydrates to fuel the body for performance, the body in a state of ketosis can just turn to stored fats instead.

Along with its fat-burning capabilities, it's also important to stress the roots of the keto diet. It was originally studied as a means to combat seizures and epilepsy in patients. This was already covered in the previous segments of this chapter. And even though there is an abundance of medication and medical treatments out there today that specifically targets epilepsy and seizures, the science still suggests that putting the body in a state of ketosis can help reduce the likelihood of seizures and epileptic episodes.

As far as accessibility is concerned, the keto diet isn't really a diet plan with food that is difficult to attain or gain access to. A lot of the food that is incorporated into a typical keto diet plan can be found in an average market or grocery store. Regardless, whether you're someone who lives in the big city or someone who comes from more rural areas, you are always going to be able to gain access to essential keto food, such as meats, eggs, nuts, cheese, and oils.

Who Isn't It For?

Again, as has already been lamented, the keto diet isn't necessarily going to be a good fit for everyone, and it's very important to determine whether you would be capable of adopting the keto diet for your own life before you actually do so. There are just certain people who are burdened with particular physical constraints that might render them incapable of adopting the keto lifestyle.

For example, it might be a little risky or dangerous for people who have a compromised gallbladder to engage in the keto diet. The reason for this is that the keto diet is one that encourages a very high consumption of fat. However, the gallbladder plays a very important role in the processing, rendering, and overall digestion of fat in the human body. Without the aid of a properly functioning gallbladder, the amount of fat taken in on a keto diet might prove to be too much for the human body to handle.

The same can also be said for people who have undergone gastric bypass or bariatric surgery. For people who undergo this kind of procedure, particularly for weight loss, it can be very difficult for the body to process the fats that it takes in. Procedures such as this can dramatically disrupt the normal metabolic functions of the body, and it can make for compromised fat metabolism.

Children and pregnant women are also discouraged from partaking in the keto diet because of the higher amount of protein requirements that they need in order to stay healthy. Individuals who are prone to kidney stones are also advised not to adopt a keto lifestyle because of the salt and fluid imbalances that arise as a result of their condition.

And lastly, people who are already underweight are also discouraged from taking on a keto diet. Remember that this is a diet that is likely to induce weight loss in a human being due to ketosis. And this can prove to be very problematic for a lot of people who already happen to be underweight or undernourished. Of course, if underweight people want to gain more weight through the keto diet, it's just a matter of raising the number of calories that they take in from fat.

CHAPTER 2:
Starting Keto

Naturally, as with any other kind of venture in life, you are always going to want to make sure that you start things off on the right foot. After all, the way that you start your keto journey is going to dramatically impact the odds of you being able to sustain it moving forward into the future or not. If you are able to start things off the right way, then it would be a lot more likely that you would be able to find results immediately. And these results would then motivate you to stay on the road that you're on. You will be able to generate momentum to help keep you going on your weight loss journey.

But if you don't start things off properly, then you run the risk of being dissatisfied with how little progress you're achieving. Then you could potentially grow discouraged from the diet, and you might end up just abandoning it altogether. And the keto diet isn't one that is going to yield the results that you want unless you actually do it properly. It's always going to have to be an all-or-nothing effort at the beginning. There can be no compromises when you're just starting out.

Of course, you aren't necessarily going to see results within the first day on a diet. It's going to take a few days or maybe even a couple of weeks for you to see results. And those initial weeks are absolutely crucial. This is precisely why this chapter is going to be fully dedicated to you doing things right even from the beginning. We are going to cover all the basic tools and principles that you need to equip yourself with for you to maximize the keto diet.

How to Start Keto

Starting a keto diet doesn't have to be so complicated. All you really need to do is keep track of the many basic rules and principles of the diet so that you would be equipped with the general guidelines that you need to make sure that you aren't doing anything wrong. And with that, here is the very first thing that you need to remember when you're starting out on the keto diet: limit the carbs!

Limit the Carbs

You can consider this to be the absolute golden rule of the keto diet. As a basic rule of thumb, you are going to want to limit your consumption of carbohydrates to around 20–30 grams every day. Getting those carbohydrate numbers down is going to be absolutely key in inducing a state of ketosis in your body. When you overindulge on your carbohydrates and you pair it with high consumption of fats, then you run the risk of gaining even more weight as time goes by. And you definitely don't want that if your ultimate goal is to burn the stored fats that you already have in your body.

Limit the Protein Intake

As counterintuitive as it might seem, it's very important that you limit your personal protein intake while you're on the keto diet. Usually, in most dietary paradigms, it is always encouraged to take in large amounts of protein to promote muscle building and metabolism. And this principle is usually true.

In the context of other dietary paradigms, high protein intake might be a good idea. However, excess consumption of protein can cause some serious stress on the kidneys. Moreover, a surplus of protein will get converted into glucose, which is something that you would want to avoid in order to trigger ketosis.

Don't Fear the Fat

Fat is something that is so often demonized in contemporary media. And to be fair, it's because we all discourage people from having excess amounts of fat in the human body. It's so easy to assume that the consumption of fat is going to make you fatter than you are. However, that is a very common misconception. Taking in an excess amount of calories than you are using to sustain your daily physical activity is what is going to induce fat and weight gain. On a keto diet, you should only ever be keeping your carbohydrates and protein intake levels constant. You should adjust your amounts of fat to meet your personal caloric needs.

Make Sure to Stay Hydrated

When you are on a keto diet, it is absolutely of the essence that you make it a point to stay hydrated *always*. As you are consuming carbohydrates, your body uses it up and converts it into energy. The excess carbohydrates that remain in your system are converted into glycogen in your liver, where they are bonded to water molecules. When you don't take in a lot of carbohydrates, your body uses this glycogen up, and that can stimulate fat burn. However, when the glycogen gets used up, all the water attached to it gets used up as well. That means that your body would be prone to getting dehydrated. As much as possible, you would want to aim for 10–14 cups of water every day while you're on the keto diet.

Load Up on Electrolytes

There are three essential electrolytes that your body needs to function properly and efficiently. These are potassium, magnesium, and sodium. We have already established that adopting a keto diet is going to put you at risk of becoming dehydrated by depleting the amount of water in your body. It's also likely that your electrolytes are going to get used up as well. And whenever there is a shortage of electrolytes in your body, you are at risk of feeling sickly. That is why you want to make sure that you are maintaining healthy amounts of electrolytes in your body while you're on this diet.

Eat Only When Necessary

When you're on the keto diet, you need to get rid of the whole mindset that tells you that you have to eat at least three to five meals every day. That's just an old dietary practice that encourages people to eat regularly in spite of busy schedules. However, when you're on the keto diet, it's very important to limit calories as much as possible. That's why it's advisable that you only ever eat whenever you're hungry. You shouldn't be forcing yourself to eat just because it's the designated eating time for the people around you.

Try to Eat Whole and Natural Foods

The whole point of the keto diet is to induce a state of ketosis while consuming only high amounts of fat, moderate amounts of protein, and limited amounts of carbohydrates. And it's true that you don't necessarily have to resort to eating only whole and natural foods to achieve a state of ketosis. It's still going to be much better for your overall health if you stick to natural and unprocessed foods. On top of natural food being healthier and having more nutrients, they are also going to help stave off cravings so that you won't be tempted to indulge in any midday snacking between large meals.

Get Your Body Moving!

Whether you are on a keto diet or not, it's very important that you still exercise. Engaging in regular physical activity isn't just going to aid in weight loss or muscle toning; it's essential in promoting overall heart health. Studies have shown that engaging in regular exercise can help strengthen your heart, lungs, muscles, and even your brain. Also, you are putting all the energy that is stored in your body to good use. Exercise can help fire up your metabolism so that you end up burning more fat, and it maximizes the ketosis that your body is going through.

Counting the Macros

Okay, so first things first: what are macros?

In order for you to understand what the typical composition of a meal should look like when you are on the keto diet, it's important that you first understand what macros are when it comes to dieting. The entire keto diet is built on the principle of consuming high amounts of fat in order to trigger ketosis in the body. To go along with the high consumption of fat, you are also going to want to make sure that you limit the amount of protein that you take in so that your body relies on stored fat for energy instead of glucose.

But you are at risk of falling into a gray area when you are merely told to eat more fat and less protein and carbohydrates. How much more is more? How much less is less? These are the questions that we're going to try to tackle within this segment of the book.

Okay, so back to the initial question at hand. What are macros? Macros are short for the word "macronutrients." The three essential macronutrients that are essential for composing an individual's daily caloric intake are protein, carbohydrates, and fats. And if you really want to make sure that you are precise and accurate in your approach to adopting the keto diet for yourself, it's very important that you are able to keep track of your macros. When it comes to ensuring the effectiveness of the keto diet, it's important that you follow your macro guidelines so that you avoid taking in too much or too little of a particular macronutrient.

And while it can be convenient to just follow a universal guideline or rubric on how your macros should be structured, it's not going to be that simple. Your macro requirements are really going to depend on the kind of lifestyle that you have. A lot of factors go into determining the amount of fat, carbohydrates, and protein that you should be taking on a daily basis. Determinants such as age, gender, physical activity, genetics, height, weight, and other facets have to come into play here. We can go into detail about how you can go about computing the proper formula you should be following for your macro intake later on. For now, you just need to understand the importance of actually keeping track of your macros while you're on a keto diet.

Once you are done with computing your ideal daily macro consumption, it all becomes a matter of you making sure that you stick to that plan so that your body enters a perpetual ketogenic state. And in order for you to sustain your state of ketosis, you are going to have to track the calories, protein, fat, and net carbohydrates that you are taking in every day. We will delve more into what net carbohydrates are in the next segment of this chapter. For now, what you have to understand is that it is essential for you to keep track of your macros so that you aren't eating in excess any of the nutrients that you are taking in.

Naturally, the more accurately you are able to track your macros, the more you would be able to discipline yourself. And the more that you are able to discipline yourself, the better the effects the keto diet will have on your system. It's only normal for you to fall off the wagon every now and then. But if you make a concerted effort to really stay on top of your macro consumption, then the more likely it will be for you to obtain the results that you want.

In order to count your macros very accurately, you might want to make use of a couple of tools to really increase the accuracy of your tracking. You can make use of a digital weighing scale for your food so that you are able to accurately measure the mass of the food that you're taking in, along with the corresponding macro values that they have. And there are also fitness apps out there, such as MyFitnessPal, that can provide you a diary or journal of your meals along with the data on macros. It might be a very tedious task, especially at the beginning, but once you get the hang of it, you're going to start to figure out how much of each macro you should be eating per meal just by merely looking at your plate. It's all just a matter of sticking to the program until you develop consistency and momentum for yourself.

Counting Net Carbohydrates

In the previous segment of this chapter, we talked about the importance of keeping track of your net carbohydrates. But what exactly are net carbohydrates, and how do you go about computing for it? It seems like there's a lot of math involved with this diet, but you're going to have to be precise if you want to maximize the effectiveness of this diet when it comes to achieving your fitness goals.

In a nutshell, net carbs are essentially the total number of carbohydrates in a particular food minus the amount of sugar alcohol and fiber within that food item. So to put things simply:

Net carbs (N) = total carbs (t) − fiber (f) − sugar alcohol (s)

You might now be thinking to yourself about what sugar alcohols are. But before we delve into that, here is a sample computation of net carbs for a medium-sized avocado.

The total carbs (t) of a medium-sized avocado would be around 17.15 grams. The fiber would measure at around 13.5 grams. The sugar alcohol in a medium avocado would be around 1.33 grams. Therefore, if we follow the $N = t - f - s$ formula, the net carbs of an avocado would be 2.32 grams.

Now, it might be important to go over what sugar alcohol levels are and why they matter in counting carbs and macros. Sugar alcohols can actually be found in all sorts of food regardless of whether they are natural, organic, or man-made. If you are someone who has a sweet tooth, then you are going to want to pay attention to the sugar alcohol levels in the food that you're eating. This is what makes a difference in whether you're going to be allowed to put a little extra honey into your tea or not.

Sugar alcohols contain some very sweet flavors that can cater to anyone's sweet tooth. They contain just about half the calories of regular sugar; however, they aren't really fully absorbed, processed, and digested by the human body. As a result, they don't really contribute to the increase in blood sugar. These are the sugars that are commonly found in food items that taste sweet and yet indicate "sugar-free" on their labels. These sweeteners are really great for

people on the keto diet but can't get rid of their sweet cravings.

There are different kinds of sugar alcohols, and some of them are going to contribute to carbohydrate levels while others won't. The sugar alcohols that do carry some carb counts will only have 50% of the total carbohydrate amounts.

For a list of sugar alcohols with or without carb counts, refer below.

Sugar alcohol with carb count:

- glycerin
- sorbitol
- isomalt
- maltitol

Sugar alcohol without carb count:

- xylitol
- mannitol
- lactitol
- monk fruit sweeteners
- erythritol

You're going to have to give up a lot of desserts and sweets if you're going to be serious about being on a keto diet and buying into this whole lifestyle. However, there are ways to circumvent these restrictions if you really need your fill of sweets. Just make sure that you don't go overboard when it comes to your net carbs and your macros. Otherwise, all of the efforts that you will put into this diet will end up being useless and moot.

But what exactly does it mean when we say that you shouldn't go overboard? If the keto diet encourages high consumption of fat, should you really be limiting yourself? Well, the short answer is yes. Move on to the next section in order to understand why and how much fat might be too much for you.

Too Much?

If you fail to be precise as you embark on your keto journey, then you will be at risk of just completely screwing everything up entirely. The margin of error while you are on the keto diet is relatively big, especially when you aren't paying attention to what you're doing or if you don't understand why you're doing it.

As we have already established in the previous segment of this chapter, fat is going to serve as the lever for your entire macro consumption structure. Your carbohydrate and protein levels of consumption should always be consistent and constant. These values and numbers should never change as long as you stay on the keto diet. All the flexibility within your diet lies in how much or how little fat you are consuming on a daily basis.

Determining the amount of fat that you need to be consuming per day is the key to you being able to meet your body's composition goals. If you are looking to lose weight, then you need to lower the amount of fat that you're taking in without increasing or decreasing your protein and carbohydrate consumption. If you want to be able to maintain the weight that you are at, then just stick to the amounts of food that you have been consistently eating. But if you're looking to gain a little weight while on the keto diet, then you're going to want to increase the amount of fat that you are taking in.

However, how much fat is too much?

That is the question that we're going to be seeking to answer in this part of the book. On a keto diet, it is always emphasized that you have to be eating large amounts of fat. However, you don't want to go overboard, because eating a surplus of calories is still going to make you gain weight even when you don't want to. It doesn't matter how little carbs or protein you consume while you're on the keto diet; if you are taking in too many calories from fat, you're still going to end up gaining weight and getting fatter. That's just how the concept of caloric deficits and surpluses work. The composition of your food doesn't really change that basic dietary principle.

Well, we are going to focus on just two different kinds of fitness and body composition goals as we try to tackle the question of how much fat is really required in a keto diet. It's practically impossible to give a definitive and singular answer to how much fat you really need to be eating because it's all dependent on what kind of goals you might have. This segment is going to touch upon two different goals.

If You Want to Lose Weight

If you are deciding to adopt the keto diet, then it's very much likely that you would fall under the category of people who are looking to lose weight. And that's not by accident. The keto diet in itself is a dietary plan that is designed to maximize weight loss and fat burn in the human body. So yes, you have decided to lose weight by consuming high amounts of fat. As contradictory as that might seem, it's actually very effective. Just make sure that you keep the following reminders to heart:

- If you are consistently losing weight at the rate of around 1–2 pounds every week, then you're definitely on the right track. Just keep on staying consistent with your macro consumption until your progress slows down or you reach a plateau.

- If you are losing just 1 pound a week, then that is okay. However, if you feel like that isn't enough, then you might want to consider cutting back on the fat that you're eating by just a little bit.

- If you are gaining weight after the length of a week, then that means you are eating *way* too much fat, and you might want to cut back significantly until you reach the point that you're actually losing weight.

- As you make your way through your weight loss journey, you will also want to pay attention to the circumference of your waistline as well. It's not just about the pounds that you lose; it's also the inches that you shed.

If You Want to Gain Muscle

Maybe you're on the skinnier side. Maybe you're a little lean and you feel like you want to be able to fill your body up a little bit more. You don't necessarily want to get fat as you try to bulk up. You want to be able to build your muscles, and you want to be able to use the keto diet to sustain yourself in the process of bodybuilding. Is it possible? Well, yes, it definitely is.

The most basic principle of building muscle in the body is making sure that you are actually taking in enough food to be able to repair your muscles from tough and strenuous workouts. And of course, you're going to have to be putting in the time and effort at the gym. You need to be engaging in anaerobic and resistance workouts that are designed to break down your muscle fibers to allow for the bodybuilding process to take place. The food that you take in is going to be used as the building blocks for your broken muscle fibers. That's essentially how you are able to build muscle without gaining fat.

However, if you are taking in too much fat in the food you eat, you might be at risk of gaining more fat along with the muscles that you're gaining as well. And if you aren't eating enough fat, you might not be getting the calories that you need to sustain your body in the midst of all your tough workouts.

Before you start working out, you are going to want to consult the keto macro formula, which will be explained later on in this chapter. The formula isn't always going to be accurate, and it definitely isn't designed to be constant. You need to be paying attention to your body and how it's responding to your daily fitness regimen. Here are a few things that you might want to keep in mind while you're building muscle on a keto diet:

• If you are gradually gaining weight with a very minimal or no increase in your waistline, then you are doing just fine. You are consuming the right amount of macros.

• If you are losing weight, then you might want to increase the amount of fat that you are eating. Also, make sure that you are eating the right amount of protein. You should be consuming around 1 gram of protein for every pound that you weigh.

• If you are gaining a lot of weight too quickly and your belly is getting larger, then cut back on the amount of fat that you are eating.

Every Person Is Different

As human beings, we are all inherently unique and different in our own ways. That's just a universal truth of human biology. No two people are ever going to be alike. Genetics and evolution have played very vital roles in shaping our bodies to be the way that they are. And as has already been emphasized in this article many times over, it's very important that people adopt a health-and-fitness regimen that is most effective for them. For some, that means taking diets that aren't based on keto principles. And for others, that means adopting keto as a lifestyle wholeheartedly.

However, not all keto lifestyles are created equal either. Just because two people say that they are both on a keto diet doesn't mean that they are both essentially eating the same kinds and amounts of food. For example, a twenty-five-year-old male bodybuilder on keto isn't going to have the same meal plan for the week as a fifty-four-year-old diabetic lady. It's always going to be different based on fitness goals and body types as well. This particular facet of this chapter will focus on how people's body types are different and why it's important to know what body type you have before you start getting into keto.

Generally speaking, there are typically only three categories of body types regardless of whether you are a man or a woman. These are endomorph, mesomorph, and ectomorph. And when we say body type, we aren't just talking about the way a person might look. We are also talking about how an individual might respond to the intake of a particular food. There are also other factors that go into determining a person's body type, such as hormonal characteristics and sympathetic nervous system (SNS) behavior. A combination of these factors has a direct correlation to the way people's inherent metabolic tendencies are structured differently. Your body type is also going to say a lot about how your body responds to exercise and dieting. That is why you really need to gain a more profound understanding of what your body type is so that you will be able to strategize your approach to dieting and training accurately. Understanding your body type is key in tailoring your keto diet program to fit your lifestyle.

However, before we go in-depth into what these three different body types are, it's important to stress that it's very rare for people to just perfectly fit into one of the three established categories. Most of the time, people are going to be a healthy mix of two or even all the body types. It's also important to note that your body type isn't going to dictate automatically how you are going to look. If you pair heavy training with strict nutrition, then it's very likely that you would end up with a toned and chiseled body regardless of what your body type is. Your body type is also going to determine the amount of protein and carbohydrate that your body would be able to tolerate before you actually start getting fat. For a more detailed description into what constitutes each body type, read on below.

Ectomorphs

To put it simply, ectomorphs are people who fall on the smaller side of the size spectrum. They are typically people who have skinny builds and lean muscles. It's also normal for ectomorphs to have longer limbs relative to the size of their torsos. These individuals typically have a very high metabolism, and they would find it difficult to gain weight and build muscle.

Think of those people in your life who can virtually just eat whatever they want while still staying trim and lean. You see them down a whole cheeseburger and a bottle of beer for dinner, and they still look like all they eat is salad greens. And while this can be seen as an advantage for a lot of people, it's definitely a problem for those who are looking to build big and sculpted muscles.

The best kind of diet program for an ectomorph would be one that focuses on high consumption of calories. And when it comes to the keto diet, they would have the most tolerance for carbohydrates. It's still important that they limit carb intake so as to induce ketosis. However, they can always make up for the caloric deficits through increased fat consumption.

When it comes to exercise, it would be better for ectomorphs to focus on strength and resistance training programs with minimal cardio. The aim is to focus on bodybuilding instead of weight loss because of their naturally high metabolic rates.

Mesomorphs

Mesomorphs are those individuals who tend to have medium-sized builds. They fall right in between ectomorphs and endomorphs. These are the people who have perceivably athletic bodies with sculpted muscles and well-defined physiques. People who are mesomorphs tend to have high levels of testosterone and growth hormones in their body's physical makeup. They are more likely to find success when it comes to promoting and stimulating muscle growth while maintaining lower levels of body fat. It's not unusual for mesomorphs to be very good at bodybuilding and strength training. However, they are still prone to gaining fat more compared to ectomorphs. That means that it's still important for them to stay mindful of the number of calories that they are taking in.

The ideal type of keto diet for a mesomorph would still be a balanced one. They are still going to have some wiggle room for carbohydrates and protein, especially when you take into consideration the fact that they are very good at building lean muscle. These muscles are going to require fuel in the form of protein and carbs. However, they are still very much prone to unhealthy weight gain, and they need to be able to moderate their food consumption appropriately. It's also likely that mesomorphs would require a lot of hydration in the form of water and electrolytes.

As far as physical training is concerned, a mesomorph would be an athlete that is well suited for resistance or anaerobic training to go along with cardiovascular or aerobic training. They are also capable of taking on heavy workout loads without having to worry about catabolism or muscle deterioration.

Endomorphs

Lastly, the endomorph is the kind of body type that would typically be indicative of a larger and more robust individual. People who are endomorphs tend to be on the bigger and stockier side. It's very easy for them to gain muscle, but it's also just as easy for them to gain fat as well. It's also very difficult for them to get rid of the fat in their bodies while maintaining their overall lean body mass. It's not unusual for endomorphs to have short torsos and limbs. It's also very likely that morbidly obese individuals are endomorphs.

However, there is a common misconception that people who are endomorphs are going to be destined to be fat and obese for the rest of their lives. That isn't the case. Regardless of anyone's body type, you are always going to be able to manipulate your behavior and your habits to stay relatively trim and lean. It's just that endomorphs are going to work much harder and stay much more disciplined compared to their mesomorph and ectomorph counterparts when it comes to staying lean.

When tailoring a keto diet around an endomorph, the emphasis really lies in calorie restriction. That means that it's very important to limit the amount of carbohydrate consumption as much as possible. It's also important to note that excess protein can be converted into glucose, which can affect the likelihood of ketosis. Endomorphs also have to make sure that they don't overindulge in the excessive

consumption of fat.

A healthy combination of endurance training, along with resistance training, can be really good for an endomorph who wants to minimize weight gain. It's very easy for an endomorph to gain muscle and fat at the same time. That is why there has to be a healthy balance between resistance workouts and cardiovascular training. Exercises that are geared more toward muscle building need to be paired with exercises that are designed for fat burning.

Keto Macro Formula

As you might have already suspected, you're going to have to be doing a lot of mathematics while you're on the keto diet. But don't worry, this is only for the first part. You won't really have to be computing with your macro formula all too often. You should only be readjusting your macros when you start losing huge amounts of weight. Typically, you would want to revisit your macro formula for every 15–20 pounds that you might lose. And the process isn't really going to be all that complicated. This segment of the chapter is going to focus on going over a step-by-step account over how you might be able to compute for your macro needs while you're on a keto diet. So get your calculators ready.

Step 1: Find Your Base Metabolic Rate (BMR)

Before you do anything else, the first computation that you are going to make is for your base metabolic rate (BMR). A BMR is essentially the average number of calories that your body is burning at a daily rate in an effort to sustain organ function and basic body processes. Take note that the BMR doesn't necessarily take into consideration the number of calories that you burn when you engage in vigorous physical activity, such as exercise. It's important to know just how many calories you are burning every day so that you would get a better idea of how many calories you need to be taking in to meet your physical composition goals.

It can be very difficult to come to a precise and accurate valuation for your BMR, but using the industry-standard Harris-Benedict equation would suffice. The computation is going to be different for men and for women.

Refer to the formula below for the computation for men:

BMR = 66 + (6.2 × your weight in pounds) + (12.7 × your height in inches) − (6.76 × your age)

Refer to the formula below for the computation for women:

BMR = 655.1 + (4.35 × your weight in pounds) + (4.7 × your height in inches) − (4.7 × your age)

There is a reason why the data listed above is required in computing for your base metabolic rate. Essentially, the more mass that you have in your body, the more calories you will need to burn in order to sustain daily bodily function. That's why there is a need to input your height and your weight. And you need to factor your age into the equation because your muscle mass gradually decreases once you go past the age of thirty. Consequently, your BMR decreases as you get older as well. Lastly, the reason why gender comes into play is that the bodies of men and women carry different metabolic needs and requirements.

Step 2: Find Your Total Daily Energy Expenditure (TDEE)

The next thing that you need to do is to find your total daily energy expenditure (TDEE). It's essentially the same as a BMR in the sense that you are computing for how many calories you are burning in a day. However, it differs because the BMR is focused primarily on the calories that your body needs to sustain vital processes only. TDEE also takes into consideration the calories that you burn as a result of the physical activity that you have within the day, particularly if you exercise. If you take your BMR and you multiply it with your level of physical activity, then you would be able to get your TDEE.

You just have to be able to classify yourself accurately to what kind of physical activity you typically have for a regular day.

- Tier 1 (minimal exercise): 1.2
- Tier 2 (light exercise for 1–3 days per week): 1.375
- Tier 3 (moderate exercise for 3–5 days per week): 1.55
- Tier 4 (hard exercise for 6–7 days per week): 1.725
- Tier 5 (intense exercise every day of the week): 1.9

Take note that exercise doesn't just necessarily mean the amount of time that you spend at the gym. You also need to take into consideration the nature of your career. If you have a profession that requires substantial physical activity, then you may consider that as a form of exercise. For example, a professional athlete, construction worker, nurse, or teacher might engage in more physical activities as compared to an accountant, computer programmer, or librarian.

Classify yourself according to the tier that best applies to you, and then multiply your BMR by the numerical value that applies to your tier. The product of that computation is going to be your TDEE.

For example, this would be the TDEE computation for an office worker with a BMR of 1,500 calories that goes to the gym three or four times a week, thereby putting them in tier 3.

TDEE = 1,500 × 1.55 = 2,325 kcal

With a base metabolic rate of 1,500 kcal, multiplied by the numerical value of 1.55, this individual's TDEE is 2,325 kcal.

Step 3: Calculate Your Body Fat Percentage

It is very important that you are able to figure out your body fat percentage so that you would also be able to figure out what your lean body mass is going to be. It's not enough that you know how much you weigh. You need to know how much of your body is composed of fat and of lean muscle. The reason this is important is, the more muscles you have, the higher the number of calories that you will be able to burn. So even if you weigh the same as another human being, you would be able to burn more calories than they do within a day if you have a lower body fat percentage.

There are a number of ways in which you can go about measuring your body fat percentage. Some of them are going to vary in terms of convenience, accessibility, and precision. Just choose the one that works best for you.

The convenient method that you can use to measure your body fat is to take a visual examination of yourself. You might not have access to complicated medical devices or instruments that would be able to give you hyper-accurate estimations of what your body fat percentage might be. You can try to take a look at yourself in the mirror or have an experienced physical trainer make a visual assessment over what your body fat percentage might be. This is not a very advisable method of measuring body fat percentage because even though it's convenient, it just doesn't offer much objectivity or accuracy. You can make use of tape measures to gauge your body fat a little more accurately, but that would still be pretty unreliable.

The actual best way for you to get an accurate body fat percentage measurement would be for you to visit a doctor's office or a physical fitness facility to get yourself assessed with the help of experts and experienced professionals.

Once you are able to get yourself measured for your body fat percentage, you would then be able to compute for your lean body mass. In a more illustrative demonstration, let's look at a man who weighs 200 pounds with 25% body fat.

In order to get his total body fat in pounds, make use of this equation:

Total body fat (pounds) = 200 pounds × 0.25 = 50 pounds

And in order to get this person's lean body mass in pounds, you would only have to subtract the total body fat from a person's overall bodyweight:

Lean body mass (pounds) = 200 pounds − 50 pounds = 150 pounds

Step 4: Calculate Your Daily Caloric Target

If your physical composition goals revolve around you just maintaining your current weight, then you don't really have to participate in this step and can move on to the next one.

If you are looking to lose weight at a gradual and healthy pace, then you're going to need to conclude each day with a caloric deficit. What that means is that you have to end up each day having expended more calories than you actually took in. Usually, a range of around 10–20% caloric deficit would induce a slow and healthy pace of weight loss for the average human being. If your goal is to have a 10% caloric deficit, then all you really need to do is multiply your TDEE by 0.10. Whatever amount you end up with should be subtracted from your TDEE, and the difference of that should be the number of calories that you should be eating every day in order to lose weight.

If you want to be able to lose weight at a more rapid pace, all you really need to do is increase the caloric deficit that you would be operating with. However, it isn't advisable for anyone to go above a 30% caloric deficit for an extended period of time.

If you are someone who is intending on packing on some more muscles, then you are going to want to have a caloric surplus. But you don't want to be eating too many calories to the point that you start packing on some unwanted fats as well. A healthy number to work with would be a 5–10% caloric surplus every day. If you are looking to have a 5% caloric surplus, then you just need to multiply your TDEE by 0.05. Take the product of that equation, and add that to your TDEE; the sum should serve as your daily caloric targets.

Step 5: Calculate Your Daily Carb Requirements

Given that this is the keto diet, you can't just be concerning yourself with the number of calories and the macros that you are consuming at any given time. In order to put your body into a ketogenic state, you are going to want to limit your carbs as much as possible. However, it would also be practically impossible to do away with carbohydrates altogether. That's why you're just going to have to compute for your daily carbohydrate requirements so that you know what you're given to work with on a daily basis.

In a ketogenic diet, you are going to want to make sure that your carbohydrates only compose around 5–10% of your daily caloric intake. We already talked about how your net carbs are essentially your total carbs minus the fiber content of these carbs. In order for you to find out just how many grams of carbs you need to be eating per day, you might want to make use of this formula:

Total carbs (grams) = TDEE (% of caloric intake) / 4

So for example, if your TDEE is 2,500 and you are looking to have your carbohydrates compose only 10% of your daily caloric intake, then your computation would look like this:

Total carbs (grams) = 2,500 (0.10) / 4 = 62.5

If this is how your computation turns out, that doesn't mean that you should automatically be shooting for 62.5 grams of carbohydrates every day. It just means that your daily carb consumption should never exceed this number so that your body won't be hindered from being in a ketogenic state.

Step 6: Calculate Your Daily Protein Requirements

The next phase of your macro computation is to determine just how much protein you should be eating on a daily basis. If your goal is to achieve ketosis, then you want to make sure that protein does not make up more than 20–25% of your daily caloric intake. It can be very easy for beginners in keto (especially bodybuilders) to make the mistake of eating too much protein.

In order for you to figure out just how much protein you need to be eating per day to stimulate muscle growth or facilitate maintenance without compromising ketosis, then you can use this segment of the book as a guide.

First of all, you are going to want to go back to step 2 and figure out what tier you fall under when it comes to your level of physical activity. If you fall under tier 1, you will want to shoot for around 0.6–0.8 grams of protein per pound of lean body mass, which you calculated in step 3. If you fall under tier 2 or tier 3, stay within the 0.8–1.0 grams per pound of lean body mass range. If you are in tier 4 or higher and especially if you engage in heavy resistance training, you are going to want to consume around 1.0–1.2 grams of protein per pound of lean body mass.

For example, if you are an average-sized female who weighs 130 pounds with around 100 pounds of lean body mass and has a rather fit and active lifestyle, then this is how you would want to go about computing your protein requirements while on keto.

You might fall under tier 4 because of the amount of training and physical activity that you partake in regularly. So that means you will want to shoot for around 1 gram of protein per pound of lean body mass that you have. That means that you are going to want to be eating around 100 grams of protein every day. That would approximately be around 400 calories of your daily caloric intake from protein.

Step 7: Calculate Your Daily Fat Requirements

And of course, within the keto diet, fats are always going to be the star of the show. As has already been touched upon, fat is going to serve as the lever in your daily food consumption while everything else should stay constant. The bulk of your meals should always be composed of fat, around 70–80% of it to be more precise. In order for you to figure out just how much fat you need to be taking in, you're just going to have to refer to this very simple formula.

Total fat percentage = 100 − total protein percentage - total carb percentage

Chances are, if you did all the computations right, you're going to end up with a relatively high number for your daily fat requirements. Don't be shocked by that. A lot of people will have a tendency to be surprised and intimidated by the amount of fat that they have to be eating while on this diet. However, you shouldn't be so scared. Achieving ketosis might feel like such a daunting and difficult task, but just go ahead and read along until the very end of this book to make the entire process easier and less intimidating for you. You might be overwhelmed with all the math that you need to do, but it's all going to be worth it once you see the effectiveness of this precision and attention to detail.

Type and Amount of Water

It should probably be a given at this point that you need to be taking in copious amounts of water regardless of whatever diet you are on. As a human being, you are going to need to fuel your body with water in order to survive and sustain yourself. It doesn't matter what kind of lifestyle you choose to live; you are going to have to make it a point to hydrate yourself religiously throughout the day. This is true if you live in places with hot climates that would cause you to sweat a lot. But this is also especially true whenever you are on the keto diet.

Any kind of diet that forces you to lower your carb intake to a minimal level is one that is going to require a very healthy consumption of water. Not a lot of people are aware that dehydration is actually one of the most common side effects that people can have whenever they start getting on the keto bandwagon. Not too many individuals are too keen about paying attention to how much water they are consuming while they are on keto. They can obsess over macros, portions, and meal plans all they want; but they should never do so at the expense of monitoring water intake. And there are perfectly rational reasons as to why water intake needs to be taken seriously while on keto.

Carbohydrates are primarily responsible for making sure that your body is always holding on to its water and sodium stores. However, when you limit the number of carbs that you take in, that means that it's easier for you to sweat out all the water and sodium that your body needs to function. That is precisely why people on keto should make it a point to drink more water than they would while on other diets.

What Type of Water Should You Be Drinking?

When we say that it's important for you to be drinking a lot of water while you're on the keto diet, we're not just talking about any kind of water. Not a lot of people would pay much attention to the amount of water they're drinking, let alone the kind of water that they're drinking. Yes, there are different kinds of water, and they all serve different purposes when it comes to hydration. And if you happen to be on the keto diet, you might want to stock up on some quality mineral water.

Sure, mineral water can be very expensive. And it's practically a luxury for most people in the world. It's not really something that you would consider to be a necessity in the keto diet. But it would make for a really good "supplement" in your efforts to hydrate yourself. If you are able to carve a little bit of space within your dietary budget for some mineral water, go ahead and invest in it.

The reason that mineral water is so good for people on keto is the fact that it serves as a really good source of calcium and magnesium. You are always going to need calcium to strengthen your bones in the body. However, it can be very hard to source calcium from your food while you're on keto, especially since dairy consumption is limited. You also need magnesium because it's an important electrolyte that you need to hydrate your muscles and prevent cramps.

Tap water is fine as a form of hydration, and if it's the only kind of water you have access to, it's not really a problem. But if you have an opportunity to stock up on valuable minerals through your water, then you should pounce on it.

How Much Water Should You Be Drinking?

The amount of water that you should be drinking is really going to vary depending on a number of circumstantial factors and variables. You need to be able to take into consideration your age, your physical activity, your body type, the climate of the place you live in, and other such things. For example, if you happen to be someone who does regular physical exercise and you live in a hot and tropical country, then you are going to want to be taking in more water as compared to someone who sits in an air-conditioned office all day.

Generally, a rule of thumb to determine whether you're hydrated or not is to ask yourself if you're thirsty. If you feel like you could drink some water at that moment, then go ahead and do so. However, it's also important that you don't excessively hydrate yourself either. Anything that is taken excessively is always going to be bad for you, even water. A good test to see whether you are staying hydrated or not is to look at the color of your pee. If you have urine that is a light yellow and is nearing the clearer side of the color spectrum, then you are well hydrated. If it is a dark yellow that is bordering on orange, then go ahead and drink a couple of cups of water right away.

If you want a numerical value on the amount of water that you have to be drinking on a daily basis, then try shooting for around ten to fourteen glasses of water a day. That should be enough to keep you feeling hydrated.

What Are Electrolytes and Why Do They Matter?

Whenever there are talks of hydration going around, it's very likely that you're going to encounter the term *electrolytes*. But what exactly are electrolytes, and how can they help you with hydration and with keto?

Electrolytes, such as magnesium, sodium, and potassium, to name a few, are important in a keto diet because they help maintain proper fluid balance within the human body. It was previously mentioned that having too much water in the body can be bad. And the reason why that is the case is that an excess of water can dilute the electrolytes that you need for your body to function in an optimal manner. This is why athletes who sweat a lot are often seen indulging in sports drinks that offer healthy doses of electrolytes.

Salt is something that is often vilified in the world of health and fitness. However, you have to understand that you need salt and sodium in your body in order for you to survive. When you don't have enough sodium in your body, it can lead to muscle cramps, fatigue, and malaise. While you are on keto, you are essentially restricting the amount of sodium in your diet because of the nature of the food that you are eating. That is why you will want to make sure that you source other alternatives for your electrolytes.

Some great low-carb options that you can source your sodium and salt from include meat broth, actual table salt, electrolyte tablets, and other such things.

What Are Some Other Alternatives for Water?

You don't always have to turn to water if you want to stay hydrated while you are on the keto diet. You are also free to hydrate yourself with tea, coffee, sparkling water, and some other liquids. According to a study, there isn't really any substantial difference between drinking water and coffee, tea, or sparkling water when it comes to hydration properties (Maughan, 2016).

CHAPTER 3:
Guide

Now that we have covered all the basic theories and principles surrounding the foundation of the keto diet, it's now time for us to go into the more practical applications of the keto diet and how you can actually adopt it into your own daily life. Visualizing your end goals is always going to be important on your path to success. But even though you always want to be keeping your eyes on the prize, it's still important that you are able to pay attention to the details that go into your efforts day in and day out.

And that's precisely what this chapter of the book is going to focus on. You are going to want to pay a lot of attention to the way that you execute and carry out your diet in your everyday life. And considering that you are a modern human being who lives a very dynamic and ever-changing lifestyle, you are going to want to have to be as versatile and adaptable as possible. You aren't always going to be eating the same food for every meal in every setting for all the days of your life. That's just plainly unsustainable and, frankly, quite sad. You are going to want to be mixing things up a little bit.

You aren't always going to be cooking things for yourself at home. Even though ideally, when you're on a strict diet, you always want to be hands-on with the food that you are eating, you can't always be overseeing every single aspect of how your meals are prepared. For example, you might not really be the most skilled person out there when it comes to the culinary arts. So naturally, you aren't always going to be able to cook your own food a few times. You are going to have to rely on outsourced meal plans, or you might even have friends or loved ones cook for you.

There will also be times when you will be forced to eat outside of the household. You have to go to work, don't you? What happens when you can't cook food for yourself and you're at the office? It would be a mistake for you not to eat, especially when you're hungry and you know that you're short on your macros. Don't worry. The keto diet is still going to be able to provide you with a lot of options for feeding even when you don't necessarily cook the food yourself.

You can even be on the keto diet while you're on vacation. The great thing about the keto diet is that it is a globally acceptable and applicable dietary paradigm. Regardless of whatever country you might find yourself in, you are always going to be able to adhere to your keto diet as long as you know what kind of food you need to be looking out for. No matter what cuisine a restaurant might specialize in, you're still going to be able to stick to your diet if you know what food you should be ordering.

The keto diet is not a very limiting or restrictive one. You don't have to live in your own kitchen for you to succeed in this diet. You just have to make sure that you adhere to certain guidelines and principles regardless of the gastronomic environment that you find yourself in. And in order to familiarize yourself with those rules and guidelines, you are going to want to take the contents of this chapter to heart. Regardless of whatever situation you end up being in, this chapter is going to help guide you through it all, even when you are thinking about cheating on your diet.

Yes, it's possible (and permissible) for you to cheat on your diet every once in a while. You can't always be so strict all the time. That's no way to live life. You don't want to be depriving yourself too much to the point that you're no longer enjoying what you're doing. Yes, you might feel yourself losing weight and becoming healthier as a result of being on this diet, but if you're not having fun while doing it or if you're completely depressed or saddened by the process, then it just isn't worth it. That's why a few cheat days here and there are always going to be permissible. But more on that later. Yes, you are going to be allowed to cheat, but there is always a proper way to go about it. And this chapter is going to help guide you through your cheat days and cheat meals as well.

As it is with any other worthwhile endeavor in life, a little guidance can always go a long way. And you should never be dismissive of any tips or lessons that anyone might be willing to impart on you. You are practically done with the crash course on learning about what the keto diet is and how it can potentially change your life for the better. You are now at the phase of actually visualizing how you are going to apply the keto diet in your own life. And this is also probably the phase in which things are going to start to get real for you.

But don't be stressed. Don't be worried. Don't be pressured at all. We're going to take things slowly and gradually. You aren't going to be bombarded by too much information that will be coming from all over the place. This chapter is going to guide you on your keto journey in a very systematic and structured manner. And what better way to kick this guide off than to start in the place where your heart rests? At home!

Keto at Home

We aren't really going to dwell too much on this segment because it should be a given at this point that the majority of your meals on keto should either be eaten or prepared at home. When you cook your own meals within the confines of your own home, you are able to pay more attention to how much you're eating and what ingredients go into your food.

Taking responsibility for your meals at home means you're actually going out and doing the grocery yourself. The best way to go about buying groceries for your stocks at home would be to come up with a meal plan that you have for yourself first. Once you know what meals you are going to be taking over the span of a week or even a month, you can visit the grocery store with specific ingredients in mind already.

Remember, if there is an option for you to purchase these ingredients in bulk, then do so. They will come out cheaper, and you won't have to keep going back to the grocery store to restock. Also, be mindful of sales or discounted items at the grocery store, especially for the food items that have lots of healthy fat. You are going to want to stock up on a lot of those items.

Generally, you are going to want to focus a lot on whole foods that have high in fat content. Stay away from processed foods as much as possible. It's not just about hitting your calorie counts or your macros. You also want to make sure that you are sourcing your macros from healthier options. For a few examples of keto essentials that you will always want to keep on your grocery list, read on below:

- low-carb vegetables (spinach, cabbage, broccoli, cauliflower, bell pepper, etc.)
- low-sugar fruits (lemon, berries, limes, tomatoes, avocados, etc.)
- seafood (tuna, shrimp, crab, mussels, cod, salmon, etc.)
- nuts and seeds (almonds, cashews, macadamias, flaxseed, pecans, pumpkin seeds, etc.)
- meat and poultry (chicken, turkey, duck, beef, venison, pork, etc.)
- eggs
- dairy (cheese, Greek yogurt, butter, heavy cream, etc.)
- olives
- oils (olive oil, avocado oil, coconut oil, MCT oil, etc.)
- coffee and tea
- condiments (mustard, sugar-free ketchup, mayonnaise, salad dressings, etc.)

Keto Outside of the House

There is this common misconception that you're just going to have to lock yourself in your house and never eat out with friends if you want to stay strict on your diet. You might dread having to go on work trips or vacations because you wouldn't know where you would have to source your meals. You are scared of the idea of having to go to a wedding party because you aren't sure if keto-friendly options are going to be served.

First of all, it's perfectly okay to have all these worries when you're on your diet. You want to stay committed and dedicated to your diet. You don't want to be messing anything up by making a few mistakes here and there. You are scared that a few bad meals are going to impede your progress and that you might undo all the hard work that you have already been putting in. It's understandable that you would feel hesitant to eat food that you didn't get to prepare yourself, especially when you've gotten used to just cooking your own meals all the time.

However, you don't have to be so hard on yourself. It's still okay for you to go out and attend social events that will require you to sit down and dine with friends. You can still go out and socialize without having to compromise your keto diet at all. It's all just a matter of you making sure that you keep a few tips in mind so that you don't end up causing too much damage to your diet.

There are a few guidelines that you are going to want to stay mindful of whenever you're eating out while on a keto diet.

Avoid Starchy and High-Carb Food

This should practically be a no-brainer at this point. The whole philosophy of the keto diet revolves around restricting carbohydrate consumption. So whenever you are browsing through a restaurant's menu, stay away from the pasta, pizza, or sandwich sections. If they start serving complimentary bread on your table, refrain from indulging in a bite. It might be difficult to stay disciplined in that scenario, but you're just going to have to restrain yourself to the best of your abilities.

Focus on Meats and Seafood

When ordering your food, try as much as possible to focus and stick to ordering just meats or seafood to compose your plate. If it's a breakfast place, maybe a few eggs might be available for your consumption as well. Load up on food that is high in fat and protein so that you won't feel tempted to indulge in the carb-heavy options.

Stick to Water for Drinks

You're at a backyard barbecue with your family, and you see all of your loved ones sipping on cold bottles of beer with their meats. Stick to water. You're at a wedding, and everyone raises a glass of champagne to toast the newlyweds. Raise your glass of water. You're at a restaurant, and someone proposes to order a bottle of wine for the entire group. Say that you'll only be having water.

It can be very easy to exceed your carbohydrate requirements by indulging a little bit too much in carb-heavy drinks. Just stay safe by sticking to water. If you want to mix things up a little bit, black coffee and unsweetened tea will be fine too.

Watch Out for Dressings, Sauces, and Spreads

Be very careful while ordering out when you're trying to stay keto-friendly. You might think that a plate of baby back ribs would be good since pork is a substance that is high in fat and protein. However, there are plenty of restaurants out there that just drown their meats in high-carb sauces, marinades, and dressings to the point that you might end up surpassing your carb requirements in a single meal. Make sure that you ask for any sauces, dressings, or spreads to be given to you on the side so that you would have better control of your portions and servings. Remember that even a tablespoon of ketchup would be enough to keep you from achieving ketosis.

Research the Restaurant Beforehand

And of course, a little research can definitely go a long way. If you already know where you're going to be eating, then that gives you an opportunity to plan out what your order is going to be. For instance, your friends might want to visit a Vietnamese restaurant in town. You can now go online and look up what Vietnamese food would be keto-friendly so that you would have a better idea of how you're going to order your food. If you're attending a wedding or a birthday party, don't be shy about asking your host or hostess what the menu is going to be. This way, you would be able to anticipate whether you would have keto-friendly options at that party or not. If keto-friendly food is not available at the event, you can opt to fill yourself up with food beforehand.

How to Cheat

Cheating. It's something that we all know is bad. A vast majority of us will agree to the fact that there is some sense of moral bankruptcy whenever people cheat. However, it would be a lie to say that none of us have ever cheated in one way or another at least once in our lives. And there's a reason that people feel an urge to cheat every so often. It's all a part of people's inherent need to achieve self-actualization. Human beings are goal-oriented creatures. And sometimes, in order to reach a certain goal, some of us will be lured into the temptation of taking shortcuts. In some cases, we are able to get what we want without really suffering any major negative repercussions. And in other cases, we end up cheating ourselves out of your own success and gratification because we decided to take the easy way out.

When you are on the keto diet, it's likely that you would have some kind of goal in mind pertaining to your fitness. Maybe you are looking to gain some muscle without really increasing your body fat. Perhaps you're seeking to lose a little more weight to save your joints from deterioration. You might be aiming to burn some belly fat so that you can fit into your old clothes. Whatever the case, the more disciplined you are with your diet, the faster you will be able to achieve your goals. And you know this by now.

However, that doesn't change the fact that you're still curious about cheating. You don't want to be on the keto diet for the rest of your life without having any occasional cheat meals, do you? There will be days wherein you will want that extra scoop of ice cream or that tasty toasted bagel with cream cheese. Does cheating on your diet every once in a while mean that you're never going to reach your goals? Well, read on to find out.

Can You Cheat?

Don't worry. Yes, you are allowed to cheat on your diet every so often. In fact, you are encouraged to cheat on your diet every once in a while. And even though that might seem like it would be counterproductive to your efforts to achieve your fitness goals, there is actually some sound reason and logic behind the occasional cheating on a diet.

Keep in mind that it isn't just your physical health that you're trying to strengthen here. You also want to make sure that you aren't compromising your mental health in the process. Cheating on your diet occasionally can actually be good for your overall outlook on dieting and health. This is because it will make it seem like your diet plan isn't so terrible and that it's actually sustainable for the long term. You can even approach your cheat meals or cheat days as rewards for sustained success. It almost incentivizes you to stay strict and disciplined for prolonged periods of time so that you are rewarded with a cheat meal in the end.

However, there are definitely some caveats to cheating as well. And that's why you are going to want to make sure that you don't overdo it with your cheat days and your cheat meals. If you cheat on a fairly regular basis, then you are at risk of just completely erasing all the progress that you make on the days that you stick to your diet. And you don't want that. You are definitely going to want to stay consistent with your diet long enough so that you will still be able to find sustained success over an extended period of time.

Just remember that the keto diet is designed to put you into a state of ketosis. However, cheating on your diet can take you out of a ketogenic state. And it's going to be very difficult for you to get back into that state once more. That is why you don't want to be so liberal with the cheat meals. As long as you stay consistent and disciplined for the most part, you should be fine.

However, you really shouldn't be beating yourself up over the occasional slip-up. You are only human after all, and you shouldn't be too hard on yourself. You are entitled to making a few bad choices here and there. As they say, having an extra slice of pizza isn't going to make you fat the same way that having just one salad isn't going to make you skinny. It's about the habitual processes that you participate in throughout your daily life that can serve as indicators of success or not.

How Often Can You Cheat?

If you are someone who is looking to build muscle, then you might be entitled to having a few more cheat days than other people who are on the keto diet. You are looking to have calorie surpluses every day after all. And even though cheating on your diet can put you at risk of gaining unwanted fat, you should still be safe for the most part as long as you keep eating clean. Ideally, if you have twenty-one meals over the course of the week, you shouldn't be having more than three cheat meals within that same span. You are going to want to stick to that ratio if you don't want to gain some unwanted flab around your belly.

However, it's a completely different story if you are someone who is actually looking to lose some weight. Yes, you are still entitled to a cheat meal every now and then. However, your cheat meals shouldn't be scheduled, and they definitely shouldn't be regularized in your diet plan. If you feel like you really need to cheat on your diet in order for it to be sustainable, then you can take an incentivized approach to it. Set a reasonable and simple goal for yourself, and only have a cheat day once you actually reach that goal. For example, a simple goal might be to lose 5 pounds. Once you lose those 5 pounds, then you would be entitled to one cheat meal. Another way you can incentivize yourself would be with the number of clean meals that you have. Try to stay disciplined for a span of 100 meals. And then treat yourself to some delicious carbs on your 101st meal before you go back to being strict and disciplined again.

Again, it's all just a matter of making sure that you are actually sticking to the diet plan for the most part. If you're inserting too many cheat meals in between, then you're practically just deluding yourself into thinking that you're getting fitter and healthier. But how much cheating can be too considered too much? This is something we can answer in the next segment.

How Much Cheating Is Too Much?

Contrary to what you might think, the answer to this question is a fairly easy one The only way that you will ever know that you're cheating too much on your diet is when you find that you're not actually making progress. It's truly as simple as that. The keto diet, if followed correctly and committedly, is going to give you positive results every time. And if you find yourself feeling frustrated at the lack of progress that you're making, then you are obviously doing it wrong. In order to avoid cheating too much on your diet to the point that you aren't really making any progress anymore, you are going to want to make sure that you never cheat so early into it. Try to stay as strict and disciplined as possible when you are just starting out. This way, you would be able to reap positive results within a relatively shorter amount of time, and then you would be able to gauge just how many cheat days you can have in your diet. Remember that the keto diet is not about deprivation. It's one that promotes holistic health. However, it should never come at the expense of a person's happiness.

CHAPTER 4:
The Pros and Cons of Keto

The duality of life is a very real concept, and it's going to apply in all aspects of existence, even dieting. Yes, there are many good aspects to going full-on keto, but there are also bad aspects, especially when people are executing it poorly or when they don't do their due diligence beforehand. It might be important for you to run through the good and the bad of keto just so you know what you're getting yourself into from a more holistic perspective. When you are able to approach the keto diet with knowledge from all angles, then that means that you are doing things right. That means you are minimizing your liabilities.

The Cons of Keto

This book has been staunchly advocating the keto diet and has been touting it as a really great dietary program for anyone to get behind. However, even though there are many benefits that come with adopting a keto lifestyle, there are still a few caveats and liabilities that you will want to educate yourself about before you really get into it.

Transition Issues

When transitioning into a keto diet for the first time, there is a tendency for people to shock their systems into developing certain flu-like symptoms, such as nausea, muscle cramps, dizziness, irritability, fatigue, and more. This is normal for a lot of people who are typically used to consuming large volumes of carbohydrates regularly. When transitioning, it might take a while for the body to acclimate itself.

Digestion Issues

One of the key elements of the keto diet is limiting the consumption of carbohydrates. And this can prove to be problematic for the digestive system because of the potential lack of fiber that you should be taking in. Fiber mostly comes from carbohydrates. And a fiber deficiency can lead to constipation, stomach pain, and other digestive issues. However, this is easily resolved through supplementation or proper meal portions.

Kidney and Liver Issues

A keto diet would prove to be very problematic for people who have liver issues. This is because the production of ketones is going to depend on the health and functionality of the liver. Putting too much stress on an already compromised liver can cause some serious complications to someone's body processes. It can also potentially cause damage to a person's kidney, especially when they are aren't hydrating properly while on keto.

Social Isolation

When you are on keto, it's always going to be helpful if you are able to surround yourself with people who understand what you are going through and will help you through it. In fact, it's more likely that you would find success in the keto diet if you have buddies who will go through this experience with you. However, a lot of the time, you're going to find yourself on the outside, looking in. This is especially going to be evident when you're dining out with friends who aren't on the keto diet. They will be ordering whatever they want, and you will be left craving for the food that they're having as well. They might be indulging in cake and ice cream while all you can do is watch them enjoy themselves.

Exhaustive Preparation and Planning

And of course, there is just no denying the amount of work and planning that goes into making sure that you are doing keto correctly. It's always going to demand a lot of your effort and your attention, particularly when it comes to meal planning and preparation. To a lot of people, the extra time that it takes to plan and prepare meals just isn't going to be worth it. There is also a lot of calculation that is involved when it comes to measuring macro requirements and caloric intakes. It might prove to be too much of a hassle for most individuals who want a simple diet that requires minimal effort.

The Pros of Keto

And while there are indeed a few cons and caveats that come with adopting the keto lifestyle, there is still a very strong case to be made for the dietary philosophy as a whole. This segment of the chapter is going to focus on the strengths of the keto diet and why the potential benefits are definitely enough to outweigh the cons.

Effective and Efficient Fat Burn

The keto diet is popularly known to be a very effective program for weight loss and fat burn. This is so because it maximizes the metabolic capabilities of the body by sourcing energy from stored fats instead of glucose. In order to achieve this, the diet limits the consumption of carbohydrates, which is a primary source of glucose, so that the body has to rely on ketones for energy to sustain itself.

Beneficial for People with Sedentary Lifestyles

In connection with the previous item on this list, the keto diet is one that definitely benefits a lot of people who live sedentary lifestyles. These days, it's so hard for people to make the time in their schedules to actually be physically active. In the advent of technological innovations, less and less physical or mechanical work is required of human beings these days. That is why there are more people who spend many hours of their daily life just sitting around or lying down. And this kind of sedentary living is a big contributor to rising obesity rates. However, the keto diet is able to induce weight loss in people even if they do lead sedentary lifestyles. Being on keto allows them to stay relatively trim even when they can't make time to go to the gym regularly.

Improved Insulin Sensitivity

The human body becomes resistant to insulin whenever it becomes overwhelmed by having to metabolize glucose and sugars that come from carbs. And insulin resistance can be bad for fat burn and weight loss because it actually slows down the body's metabolic capacity. Insulin resistance is particularly disadvantageous to athletes because it can weaken a person's athletic performance. However, being on the keto diet minimizes a person's risk or exposure to insulin resistance due to the restriction of glucose and carbohydrate consumption.

Delicious Dieting

You have probably encountered a few people in your life who start diets that last only a week and then go back to their unhealthy eating habits. That's because their ideas of dieting is to eat bland chicken breasts and boring garden salads always. When you don't add life or flavor to the food that you eat, it's very unlikely that you will be happy, and that's why the keto diet is really easy to get behind. It doesn't really restrict flavor at all. It's a diet that promotes the increased consumption of fats, and some of the most delicious food in the world have high fat content.

Accessible Dieting

One of the major hesitations that people have before they enroll in certain diet programs is that they can be very difficult to sustain.

And these diets become difficult to sustain because either they can get really expensive or the food can be really hard to source. However, these are two things that one wouldn't really have to worry about while on the keto diet. It still promotes regular eating, albeit with a few tweaks to the portioning of this food. There really isn't any special food out there that is required to succeed at the keto diet. It's all just a matter of scaling and proper adaptation.

Research-Based Philosophy

And of course, one of the major pros of the keto diet is the fact that it is a diet that is backed by heavy research and scientific studies. It's not just some fad that has recently sprouted up without any real backing or substance. This is a dietary paradigm and philosophy that has undergone rigorous scrutiny, criticism, study, analysis, and experimentation. The principles that the keto diet is founded on are actually seeded in science and not just speculation. The pros of the keto diet have been proven by experts and practitioners in the science and fitness sectors time and time again.

CHAPTER 5:
Usual Mistakes

Don't feel bad about making a few mistakes here and there when you are embarking on your keto journey. This is especially going to be true at the start when you're just trying to get the ball rolling and establish a rhythm with your new routine. There are so many people who start off with their diets filled with a lot of hope and optimism. They are expecting the best, and they believe that they are so excited about the progress that they will make while they're on their diets.

However, these same people might find themselves maybe two, three, or four weeks down the line feeling frustrated and disappointed at the lack of progress they are making. They feel incredibly discouraged at how their efforts aren't paying off, and they will be tempted to abandon their diets altogether. This is something that happens all too often, and it's always unfortunate whenever people just give up at the first signs of difficulty or inconvenience.

You have to keep in mind that in dieting—and life in general—it's okay to make mistakes. Mistakes are a very normal aspect of human existence. What isn't okay is *not* taking your mistakes and learning from them as you move forward into the future. Whenever you stumble and fall as you're making your way through your fitness journey, it's important to remind yourself that not all is lost. Making just one mistake doesn't make you a complete failure.

However, prevention is still better than a cure. You want to give yourself room to make some mistakes, especially in the novice stages. But you might also want to try to avoid these mistakes altogether. And that's exactly what this chapter is designed to help you out with. Instead of waiting for you to make your mistakes and learn from them, this chapter is going to give you insight into some usual mistakes that you are prone to making while you're on this diet.

If you are able to anticipate making these mistakes, then you would be in a better position to avoid committing them. So you need to be paying close attention to the way that you are conducting yourself in your diet. You need to be able to police yourself and make sure that you are doing things the right way.

What Are the Usual Mistakes People Make on Keto?

You Aren't Eating Enough Fat

When you are just beginning your keto journey, it can be very easy to become shocked at the amount of fat that you will have to be consuming for your meals. The keto diet is truly a unique and revolutionary diet in the sense that it calls for a seemingly inordinate amount of fat to be consumed on a regular basis. Most people aren't used to eating the amount of fat that they're eating while on a keto diet. It can be very easy to cut back a little bit on those fats because your instincts tell you that they're just too much. However, if this persists, you run the risk of not getting enough calories from fat to make your diet a sustainable one.

You Are Consuming Too Much Protein

The keto diet is not a high-protein diet. A lot of athletes, especially those who engage in some kind of strength or resistance training, are going to rely on protein for muscle stimulation and growth. However, on the keto diet, the consumption of protein is limited to a certain degree. If you are on the keto diet, you can't be overindulging on protein because this can be counterproductive to the intentions of the ketosis. When there is an excess of protein in the body, it gets converted into glucose. And what ends up happening is that your body relies on that glucose for energy instead of your stored fats.

You Are Taking in Too Many Calories

The keto diet is one that encourages the high consumption of fat for every meal, and at the same time, it is a diet that is designed to stimulate weight loss and fat burn. However, people still need to understand the basic formula of weight gain. You always need to make sure that your caloric expenditure is more than your caloric intake. This means that you shouldn't be eating more calories than you are using up to go about your daily life, and it can be very easy to go on caloric surpluses on a keto diet because fats are typically calorically dense foods. This is why macro documentation and counting are always optimal.

You Aren't Keeping Yourself Hydrated

There is no way that your body would be able to maximize its fat-burning capacity if you're not taking enough water during the day to sustain you. Hydration is always going to be important for any bodily function. Studies have shown that water makes up approximately 60% of the human body. If your body is struggling to keep itself hydrated, there is a good chance that it won't be able to conduct basic body processes properly, such as burning fat.

You Aren't Restocking on Electrolytes

It's not really all that rare for people to experience flu-like symptoms when they make that initial transition into the keto lifestyle. This happens because when the body is caught in a prolonged state of ketosis, the brain might end up running on very low energy because the body is still learning to source its fuel from stored fats. As a result, people can experience lightheadedness and occasional dizziness as well. This is often referred to as the keto flu.

That's why electrolytes can really come in handy in the keto diet's initial phases. When you get a healthy dose of electrolytes, you are able to alleviate these flu-like symptoms more effectively.

You Are Taking in Too Much Dairy

You might be surprised to know that there are so many people in the world who actually have lactose intolerance. Some people might just have very mild cases of lactose intolerance to the point that they don't really feel or notice it. However, one of the effects of taking in dairy when you are lactose intolerant is that it can prevent you from losing weight. Dairy can actually have inflammatory properties for certain people, and that can completely compromise the entire weight loss process.

You Indulge in Too Many Snacks

Again, it's very important to stress the key role that macro counting and food journaling is going to play in your keto lifestyle. It can be very easy to assume that you will be losing weight if you stick to just eating high amounts of fats. However, if you overindulge, you are still going to end up gaining weight. This is especially true if you are a frequent snacker. You might think that you aren't taking in enough calories because you cut down on portions during your big meals. However, you can quickly gain all those calories back if you keep on snacking throughout the day in between your large meals.

You Eat Food That Has Secret Carbs

You need to stay mindful always of the composition of the food that you eat. That's why it's always safest for you to be the one who actually prepares and cooks your food. However, if you're not necessarily skilled in the culinary department, you might have to rely on other people's cooking or ready-made meals for sustenance. And this can be problematic because you might not know that certain food items carry a lot of secret carbohydrates. For instance, breaded pork chops might seem like an acceptable food on the keto diet. However, the breading that is used for those chops can carry a lot of carbohydrates that would prevent your body from achieving ketosis.

You Don't Get Enough Sleep at Night

In your efforts to lose weight, it's always important that you get some quality sleep at night. If you aren't sleeping enough, then you are essentially putting your body through more stress and tension. As a result, your body is going to slow down its metabolic rate in an effort to retain fat as a form of precautionary measure in case you need extra energy during times of extreme stress. Also, sleeps help repair muscle fibers that are broken when you engage in rigorous training and fitness regimens. You should always be looking to get some extra z's when you're on the keto diet.

You Obsess over the Number on Your Weighing Scale

As you are trying to lose weight, it can be very easy to become a slave to that weighing scale of yours. You might obsess over the numbers on the scale to the point that you actually measure your weight multiple times in a day. And that's always dangerous. There will be instances wherein you won't be losing weight even though you are burning a lot of fat. This is especially true if you are building muscle through resistance training and strength workouts. Remember that muscles weigh more than fat. And even though you're burning a lot of fat, you might still be maintaining the same weight because you're gaining muscles as well in the process.

You Are Eating All the Wrong Kinds of Fats

Just because the keto diet is a dietary principle that encourages the high consumption of fats doesn't mean that you should get free rein over all fatty foods. There is still such a thing as bad fats, such as the fat that comes from junk and processed foods. You want to make sure that you are sourcing your fat from quality whole foods that are all natural and nutritionally dense. The fat that you get from a cup of processed vegetable oil isn't going to be the same as the healthy fat that you can get from an avocado.

You Don't Plan Your Meals Ahead of Time

Meal planning is always going to be key in any kind of diet. Whether you're on keto on or not, meal planning can really go a long way in making sure that you are meeting your goals and staying on the path that you have laid out for yourself. When you plan out your meals, it saves you the stress and trouble of having to think about what your next meal is going to be or where it's going to come from. It can help prevent you from making any rash decisions that might end up compromising your diet.

You Expect Immediate Results

You should always make sure that you never expect instant gratification whenever you are just starting out on your fitness journey. It can be very easy to get discouraged and sad whenever you step on the weighing scale within that first week and see that you haven't made much progress. That's just not how fitness and wellness works. It's not something that you can just take part in and expect immediate dramatic results. It's always a gradual and incremental improvement that you need to invest in. That's why it's important to pay attention to all your little habits and the health choices that you make throughout the day because they can really add up.

You Compare Your Progress to Those of Others

Whatever happens to you on your fitness journey is your own business, and it shouldn't be anyone else's. You need to take full ownership of whatever progress you make, and you always need to be proud of all your milestones regardless of whether they are big or small. You can't be discouraged just because you see someone else losing more weight than you are. That's just not how fitness works. Everyone has different body types, lifestyles, circumstances, and dispositions. Focus on your own path and on your own progress. You shouldn't be comparing yourself to other people.

You Don't Ask for Help and Guidance

It's always going to be okay to ask for help whenever you need it. You should never be too proud or conceited to think that you already know everything on your journey to health and wellness. There is always going to be something new to learn. And you should never close your mind to these opportunities to gather new information or data that would be able to help you reach your goals. Don't be so naive as to think that you are capable of doing everything on your own.

You Prioritize Macro Counting over Quality Control

It's not just all about the macros. Yes, you are always going to want to obsess over the numbers so as to achieve accuracy and precision in your keto lifestyle. However, your macro counting should never come at the expense of the quality of food that you eat. For example, you might think that in order for you to meet your daily requirements for fat, you should down a cup of olive oil. That isn't going to be very smart because it's not quality eating. You're reaching your macros, but your tummy won't be happy.

You Indulge in Too Many Cheat Meals

It might be okay to indulge in a cheat meal or a cheat day every once in a while when you are on the keto diet. This is something that we have already discussed in an earlier chapter of the book. Cheating can be very beneficial, especially with regard to your overall mental outlook and emotional well-being. However, if you indulge in one too many cheat meals, then it's going to end up balancing out all the progress that you've made when you actually follow the diet plan.

CHAPTER 6:
Supplementation

One important topic that we're going to have to cover as we're discussing diets and fitness regimens is supplementation. When you are conscious about your health and your fitness, you are always going to want to do whatever it takes to gain an edge. And sometimes, that means resorting to various supplements that you can take to maximize your health and fitness efforts further. However, in the context of the keto diet, wherein a lot of things are restricted and limited, is it okay to be dabbling into supplements?

Before we delve into answering that question, it might be important to establish first what supplements are and how they fit into the world of health and wellness.

A dietary supplement, also referred to as food supplement or nutritional supplement, is an item that can be ingested to deliver certain nutrients that might otherwise not be consumed in sufficient quantities. Examples of these food supplements could be amino acids, fatty acids, vitamins, minerals, and other such substances. A lot of the time, these supplements will come in the form of tablets, capsules, liquids, pills, or powders.

There are many debates that rage on in various forums and platforms surrounding the necessity of supplements in a person's daily life. But a lot of these debates are moot in the context of this book. The only thing that you need to interest yourself in is whether supplementation would be good for you on your keto journey or not. And if it is going to be good for you, it's important that you know the degrees and forms of supplementation that you will need to incorporate into your regimen.

That is precisely what this chapter is going to try to help you out with and guide you through. Supplementation doesn't really have to be a very complicated facet of dieting. However, if you want to be very serious in your approach to dieting, then it might be necessary to develop a deeper and more profound understanding of supplementation within the context of the keto diet.

Do You Need to Supplement Keto?

If you're looking for the CliffsNotes version of the answer to this question, it's no. You don't really need to be engaging in supplements while you are on keto. The truth is that as long as you're paying a lot of attention to the food that you eat and you are able to meet your macros accordingly, then there really isn't going to be any need for you to resort to the use of supplements at all. However, that doesn't mean that you should just completely shut yourself off to the prospect of incorporating supplements into your health regimen.

While it's true that you don't really *need* supplements in order for you to succeed at the keto lifestyle, it is also true that supplements can make it a lot easier for you to actually meet your nutrient goals and targets. You may consider supplements to be dietary luxuries that offer convenience and ease while you are pursuing your keto goals. This is especially going to come in handy when you aren't going to be used to the idea of shoveling large portions of food that is rich in fat down your throat all the time. The truth is that a lot of people often get surprised at how much fat they need to be eating to be on keto. And sometimes, they're just going to need a little help in the form of supplements.

Also, it's important to note that transitioning into the keto diet is no small ordeal. The keto diet is a very transformational one in the sense that it completely turns your entire metabolic system on its head. And whenever that's the case, people might end up feeling overwhelmed at all the changes that are taking place in their bodies. This is why some individuals might even experience what is referred to as the keto flu. And there are going to be certain supplements that can actually aid in counteracting the symptoms of the keto flu.

The keto diet is also one that discourages the intake of carbohydrates, and that might mean a minimal consumption of fruits and vegetables, which offer a lot of nutritional value. Keto practitioners can make use of pills, capsules, or tablets that contain these valuable vitamins and minerals that they would typically obtain from fruits and vegetables. These supplements can help fill in the nutritional gaps that a person might need.

If you feel like it would do you a lot of good to take in some supplements while you're on keto, then go ahead and read on until the very end of this chapter. But if you feel like you would be able to meet all your nutritional needs on keto even without resorting to the use of supplements, just read the rest of the chapter anyway. You never know what lessons you might pick up along the way. You have nothing to lose and everything to gain by feeding yourself with more knowledge.

What Supplements Do You Need When You're Doing Keto?

So you've taken an interest in the kinds of supplements that would be able to help make your keto journey easier and more effective. Then you've come to the right place. This segment of the chapter is going to help brief you on what kinds of supplements you need to be looking out for when you should be taking these supplements and how much of these supplements you should regularly be taking.

Just like you do with your macros from real food, you will want to make sure that you pay close attention to the supplements that you are taking in. You don't want to put yourself at risk of actually compromising the ketosis in your body just because you were too careless in your approach to supplementation. Again, when it comes to finding success in any fitness regimen, especially the keto diet, attention to detail is always going to be of the essence.

Electrolytes

There's no point in concealing the fact that being on a very strict keto diet might result in people avoiding typical foods that are rich in electrolytes, such as sodium, magnesium, calcium, and potassium. And if you don't load up on these electrolytes, your body wouldn't really be able to perform at an optimal level. Whenever you go on any kind of low-carb diet, such as the keto diet, your kidneys are going to end up dumping a lot more water than usual. And along with that water, you will be losing sodium and other electrolytes that you're going to need to replenish.

If you don't have enough sodium or potassium in your system, it could result in the development of headaches, nausea, fatigue, and even constipation. Again, during the initial phases of keto, these symptoms are often indicative of what is referred to as the keto flu. If you are going on the keto diet, partaking in supplements that are rich in electrolytes can help alleviate the symptoms that come with keto flu.

To go more in-depth with the kinds of electrolytes that you need to be paying attention to when you want to supplement your keto diet, just remember these four basic ones: sodium, magnesium, potassium, and calcium. Sodium helps retain water in your system, and it also aids in basic muscle function. Ideally, you will want to be consuming around 2,300 milligrams of sodium per day.

Magnesium is an electrolyte that is primarily responsible for promoting heart health, immunity, and proper muscle function. You should be looking to take in 350–450 milligrams of magnesium every day. Potassium is an electrolyte that helps in regulating blood pressure and heart rates. It also happens to aid in fluid balance. You should be shooting for around 4,700 milligrams of potassium each day. Lastly, calcium is an electrolyte that is popularly known to strengthen bones and joints. However, it also aids in muscle contraction and healthy blood clotting. It's advisable for both men and women to be taking in 1 gram of calcium per day.

Clean Protein

The keto diet is one that prioritizes the consumption of fat over the other macronutrients. However, protein is never something that you want to disregard, especially if you are one who lives a relatively active and physically demanding lifestyle. We already touched on the amount of protein that you should be consuming every day in a previous chapter of this book. It's all dependent on your lean body mass, body fat percentage, and TDEE. And even though the keto diet only allows for moderate consumption of protein, the requirements can still get pretty high.

Protein is important for building muscle and promoting immune health. If you feel like you are having trouble with meeting your daily protein requirements, it might be good to resort to some clean protein sources to help you get those numbers up. Whey or plant-based protein powders can serve as great supplements to help you achieve your protein intake goals.

Vitamin D

Vitamin D is a very complex nutrient because it functions as both a vitamin and a hormone. It is a very powerful nutrient health-wise, and it really does a great deal to affect the body's overall health positively. However, it can be very hard to source healthy doses of vitamin D from food alone. Vitamin is responsible for promoting bone density, muscle health, strength retention, and immune system health. It also aids in the absorption of electrolytes and other minerals.

As far as supplementation dosage is concerned, you should aim for around 400 international units of vitamin D every day.

MCT Oil

MCT, or *medium-chain triglyceride*, is a type of fat that is utilized as energy immediately to support physical activity instead of being stored as fat. Essentially, MCT oil is the kind of fat that is designed to induce a ketogenic state in the body. Usually, you can find MCT in coconut oil, cheese, butter, yogurt, and others. However, these foods can be relatively high in calories, and they also carry other macros, such as carbs and proteins. It's possible for you to take more concentrated doses of MCT oil so that you don't have to deal with all the extra *fat*, so to speak.

Omega-3 Fatty Acids

Omega-3 fatty acids are great forms of fat that can offer great nutritional value for any kind of dietary regimen. The fatty acids eicosapentaenoic acid (EPA) and docosahexaenoic acid (DHA) are known to anti-inflammatory acids. They also help reduce a person's risk and exposure to heart-related problems and mental deterioration.

When you are on a high-fat diet like keto, you are exposing yourself to the overconsumption of omega-6 fatty acids. These are the kinds of fats that you would typically find in processed vegetable oils and canned goods. When there is an imbalance in your body that favors omega-6 fatty acids, you are prone to contracting many inflammatory diseases. The consumption of omega-3 fatty acids would be able to offset and balance out your consumption of omega-6 fatty acids.

Exogenous Ketones

When your body goes into a state of ketosis, the liver produces ketones, which are then converted into energy instead of glucose. However, you don't always have to rely on your liver to be the only source you have for ketones. There is a way for you to ingest more ketones from external supplements. These are called exogenous ketones. These supplements are designed to help your body reach ketosis at a faster rate, but they also have other health benefits too. These supplements are also known to aid in overall athletic performance by promoting muscle health and recovery. They are also known to help in curbing people's appetites so as to prevent unnecessary snacking.

Caffeine

While most people wouldn't really consider their morning cup of coffee to be a supplement, the caffeine that you get from your coffee certainly helps your body function optimally throughout the day. Caffeine is responsible for people who require natural sources of energy and focus. It is also known to aid in boosting a person's overall athletic performance. This can be a very useful supplement for people on the keto diet who are looking for quick pick-me-ups minus the calories and weight of other macronutrients.

CHAPTER 7:
Keto Compared to Other Diets

Again, the keto diet isn't the only diet that exists in the world of fitness and wellness. You are afforded a wide range of options and methodologies that you can choose to adopt for yourself. This kind of variety and diversity within the industry of dieting is always going to be good. This way, people are going to be able to find the diet that best suits their own personal needs and their own lifestyles. And if you are one who is contemplating adopting the keto diet for your own life, then you're going to want to know just how it compares to other alternatives.

And that is going to serve as the topic for this chapter. You are going to be given a glimpse into what the keto diet really is and how it stacks up relative to the other popular diets out there on the market. This kind of comparative analysis would be able to do two things. One, it will allow you to gather perspective on the diet industry and the variety of options that are available for you to try. And two, it will offer you a more informed opinion and a stronger resolve for whatever diet plan you do eventually choose to adopt for yourself in the future.

A Case for Keto Being the Best Diet Plan Out There

It's true that there are indeed countless diet plans out there on the market, and it would be too arrogant to say that the keto diet is the best among them all. However, it would be fair to say that the keto diet is the best one for you *personally* if it happens to serve your needs and your goals more effectively.

The keto diet is a low-carb diet that is designed to put the human body into a heightened ketogenic state, which would inevitably lead to more pronounced fat burn and weight loss. It is a fairly accessible diet with a lot of keto-friendly foods being readily available in market places at relatively affordable prices. It isn't really a diet that is reserved only for the affluent and elite.

As far as effectiveness is concerned, there is just no denying how impactful a keto diet can be for a person who wants to lose a drastic amount of weight in a healthy and controlled manner. The keto diet also enforces discipline and precision for the agent by incorporating macro counting and food journaling so as to ensure accuracy and accountability in the diet. There are no external factors that can impact how effective this diet can be for you. Everything is all within your control.

And lastly, it's a fairly sustainable diet plan, given that it doesn't really compromise on flavor or variety. Sure, there are plenty of restrictions. But ultimately, there are a lot of alternatives and workarounds that can help stave off cravings. If all these principles and reasons apply to you and your own life, then it would definitely be safe to say that the keto diet is the best one *for you*.

What Sets Keto Apart from Others?

But how exactly does keto stack up against other diet plans out there? Well, if your purpose for dieting is weight loss, then it would be prudent to look into other diets that are similar to the keto diet's goals of inducing weight loss and fat burn. You should gain a better understanding of these diets and why the keto diet would probably still be the better one for you. The three diets that are most commonly compared to the keto diet in terms of food composition and physical effects are Atkins, paleo, and Whole30.

Atkins

The Atkins and keto diets are so similar in the sense that they both promote high consumption of fats, moderate consumption of protein, and minimal consumption of carbohydrates. Typically, while on Atkins, a person's typical diet would be composed of 60% fat, 30% protein, and 10% carbohydrates. This is still a relatively minimal carbohydrate composition even when you take into consideration the keto breakdown of 75% fat, 20% protein, and 5% carbohydrates.

The problem with Atkins isn't really found in the higher carbohydrate consumption. It's mostly found in the elevated consumption of protein. Any excess protein that the body doesn't use up for muscle building or repair is converted into glucose. And that glucose is going to be used for energy instead of the stored fats that you can have, hereby making the metabolic rate of your body slower. The keto diet still offers you the protein benefits of building and repairing muscles without compromising the benefits of ketosis at the same time.

Paleo

The paleo diet is one that is gaining vast popularity in the contemporary fitness industry. It stems from the studied dietary practices of the Paleolithic era, which was dependent on the hunter-gatherer system of food rationing and production. It is a diet that focuses wholly on whole foods that are free from any processing. Food items such as wheat, grains, dairy, legumes, processed sugars, processed oils, corn, processed fat, and the like are prohibited. It focuses on the high consumption of meats and non-starchy vegetables.

Like the keto diet, the paleo diet also happens to be a low-carb diet that emphasizes a higher consumption of fats and proteins. However, it doesn't really limit the number of carbohydrates or calories that a person might take on a daily basis. It's a diet plan that focuses entirely on the composition of food without the quantity of it, and that can be problematic for a lot of people who have very specific physical composition goals.

Whole30

Whole30 is essentially a stricter version of the paleo diet. It is a diet plan that is essentially structured as a thirty-day program of strict eating under paleo principles. It completely eliminates the consumption of processed foods, starchy vegetables and carbohydrates, sweeteners, dairy products, legumes, and more. Once the thirty-day period is over, you are then advised to reintroduce certain food groups gradually in your diet and observe what kind of effect or impact these can have on you. This is how you will be able to find out what kind of food you have a general intolerance to.

However, the Whole30 diet doesn't really factor in macro counting and calorie counting either. That means that people on the Whole30 diet are still susceptible to gaining weight and getting fat in spite of the restrictive nature of the diet.

These might only be three examples of similar dietary programs and methodologies, and there are so many other diets out there that the keto diet can actually be compared to. However, that would probably make for another book entirely. The point that this chapter is merely trying to make and emphasize is that there are always going to be certain caveats in any kind of dietary philosophy. There will be benefits, and there will be cons as well. The best kind of diet isn't the one that every single person in the world is going to find success in. Rather, it's the one that is going to enable you to reach all your own personal fitness goals and dreams. And it would be very hard to deny the fact that the keto diet manages to do precisely that for so many different kinds of people in the world.

CHAPTER 8:
Beginner Keto Meal Plan

You have now been briefed on various foundational aspects of the keto lifestyle. You now understand what it is, what it hopes to achieve, and what basic principles you need to be able to abide by in order to yield the results that you want. You have also familiarized yourself with the science behind why it's an effective diet plan and why it can prove to be beneficial in your weight loss or fitness goals. You've already been briefed on the basic principles and guidelines that you need to stick to when you're just starting out on your keto journey, and you've also been taught how to break through whatever plateaus you might encounter along the way.

We talked about how there are different body types for every individual and how the keto diet might yield different responses from these particular body types. You've also been taught about how you need to factor in exercise and training into your keto lifestyle and how these two concepts should go hand in hand with each other. You've been taught how to calculate your macros and your nutritional needs for your daily food intake.

In chapter 3, we talked about how you can still subscribe to keto dining principles regardless of where you are. We've also touched on the concept of cheat days and whether or not you should be cheating on your diet every so often. You've also been briefed on the basic food that keto practitioners turn to in order to define and compose their meal plans. We also discussed the best possible food combinations to maximize both taste and overall nutritional wellness. You have been taught about the "dangers" and potential pitfalls of doing the wrong kind of keto, and you have also been briefed on some common mistakes that you might be prone to making while you are on this diet program.

We also looked into whether or not you should be incorporating the use of nutritional supplements while you are on the keto diet. We discussed how different fitness goals might require different forms and degrees for supplementation here and there. We also discussed how the keto diet has managed to set itself apart from other dietary philosophies and paradigms.

But this chapter, in particular, is going to focus on the basics of the diet—the actual food. Enough with the theory. Let's go to actual visual representations of the keto diet and tangible ideas that you can adopt for your own personal meal plans as well. Again, as has already been mentioned in previous chapters, the way that you are going to structure your meal plan really is dependent on the type of body and lifestyle that you already have.

In this chapter, we are going to be providing a sample meal plan that will span the course of three days for two different kinds of people. The first meal plan is designed for an overweight adult male who struggles with burning fat. The second meal is designed for an average-sized female woman who tries to stay relatively active in her daily life.

Sample Three-Day Meal Plan for an Overweight Male Adult

Biologically speaking, males have a tendency to burn more calories on a daily basis as compared to their female counterparts. However, that doesn't mean that females are prone to being fatter. Men are still prone to becoming fat, especially those who are categorized under the endomorph body type. Whenever this is the case, it's important to put an emphasis on minimal consumption of carbohydrates and protein. The emphasis needs to be on the moderate to high amount of fat consumption depending on that individual's daily caloric expenditure.

This is a sample three-day meal plan for an overweight male adult. If you notice, the follower of this meal plan is still going to be subjected to a relatively high number of calories. However, if you take into consideration the BMR of an overweight male adult, it's going to be significantly much higher than a skinny male adult. That's why there will be a more liberal allowance of calories as long as the ketogenic properties of the diet are not compromised.

Day 1

Breakfast: Bunless cheddar cheeseburger with salad greens and Thousand Island dressing

- Primary ingredients:
- 1 medium-sized egg
- 75 grams of ground pork
- 1 slice of American cheddar cheese
- 1 ounce of tomatoes
- 1 tablespoon of butter
- 30 grams of cucumbers
- 30 grams of lettuce
- 1 tablespoon of olive oil
- 1 tablespoon of mayonnaise dressing
- Calories: 693 kcal
- Macros:
- Total fat: 62 grams
  - Saturated fats: 23 grams
  - Monounsaturated fats: 24 grams
  - Polyunsaturated fats: 5 grams
- Carbohydrates: 5 grams
  - Fiber: 1 gram

- ○ Carbs from sugar: 2 grams
- Protein: 33 grams

Lunch: Zucchini and beef lasagna in Alfredo sauce
- ➤ Primary ingredients:
- 1 tablespoon of salted butter
- ¼ cup of sliced zucchini
- 1 tablespoon of olive oil
- 75 grams of 75% lean ground beef
- 25 grams of cheddar cheese
- 10 milliliter of heavy cream
- ➤ Calories: 569 kcal
- ➤ Macros:
- Total fat: 54 grams
- ○ Saturated fats: 22 grams
- ○ Monounsaturated fats: 13 grams
- ○ Polyunsaturated fats: 2 grams
- Carbohydrates: 4 grams
- ○ Fiber: 0 grams
- ○ Carbs from sugar: 1 gram
- Protein: 17 grams

Dinner: Creamy spinach, artichoke, chicken, and vegetables
- ➤ Primary ingredients:
- 1 tablespoon of olive oil
- 5 grams of artichokes

- 25 grams of cheddar cheese
- 2 grams of raw spinach
- 80 grams of chicken thigh with skin
- 30 grams of romaine lettuce
- Calories: 527 kcal
- Macros:
- Total fat: 46 grams
  - Saturated fats: 9 grams
  - Monounsaturated fats: 15 grams
  - Polyunsaturated fats: 4 grams
- Carbohydrates: 6 grams
  - Fiber: 0 grams
  - Carbs from sugar: 0 gram
- Protein: 26 grams

Day 2

Breakfast: Spam-and-cauliflower casserole

- Primary ingredients:
- 1 tablespoon of olive oil
- ½ cup of raw cauliflower
- 50 milliliter of all-purpose cream
- 50 grams of cheddar cheese
- Calories: 587 kcal
- Macros:
- Total fat: 53 grams

- ○ Saturated fats: 18 grams
- ○ Monounsaturated fats: 10 grams
- ○ Polyunsaturated fats: 1 gram
- Carbohydrates: 5 grams
- ○ Fiber: 1 gram
- ○ Carbs from sugar: 4 grams
- Protein: 16 grams

Lunch: Pork chop satay with mixed vegetables and peanut sauce
- ➢ Primary ingredients:
- 1 tablespoon of salted butter
- 1 tablespoon of olive oil
- 50 grams of raw broccoli
- ½ ounce of peanuts
- 75 grams of sliced pork belly
- ➢ Calories: 560 kcal
- ➢ Macros:
- Total fat: 52 grams
- ○ Saturated fats: 16 grams
- ○ Monounsaturated fats: 21 grams
- ○ Polyunsaturated fats: 12 grams
- Carbohydrates: 4 grams
- ○ Fiber: 3 grams
- ○ Carbs from sugar: 1 gram
- Protein: 20 grams

Dinner: Grilled-chicken Caesar salad

- ➢ Primary ingredients:
- 1 tablespoon of olive oil
- 50 grams of unpeeled cucumber
- ½ cup of shredded lettuce
- 1 tablespoon of Parmesan cheese
- 2 slices of Caesar bacon
- 75 grams of grilled chicken
- ➢ Calories: 541 kcal
- ➢ Macros:
- Total fat: 47 grams
  - Saturated fats: 4 grams
  - Monounsaturated fats: 10 grams
  - Polyunsaturated fats 1 gram
- Carbohydrates: 5 grams
  - Fiber: 0 grams
  - Carbs from sugar: 2 grams
- Protein: 23 grams

Day 3

Breakfast: Bacon bombs in blue cheese dressing and buttered veggies

- ➢ Primary ingredients:
- 1 tablespoon of olive oil
- 1 tablespoon of salted butter
- 75 grams of raw cauliflower

- 75 grams of lean ground pork
- 1 slice of bacon
- 2 tablespoon blue cheese dressing
➤ Calories: 542 kcal
➤ Macros:
- Total fat: 48 grams
  - Saturated fats: 10 grams
  - Monounsaturated fats: 14 grams
  - Polyunsaturated fats: 2 grams
- Carbohydrates: 5 grams
  - Fiber: 2 grams
  - Carbs from sugar: 3 grams
- Protein: 25 grams

Lunch: Fish patty with pork rind, side greens, and avocado mayo

➤ Primary ingredients:
- 1 tablespoon of olive oil
- 1 tablespoon of avocado oil
- 10 grams of pork rinds
- 75 grams of cooked salmon
- ½ cup shredded lettuce
- 1 tablespoon of mayonnaise

➤ Calories: 547 kcal
➤ Macros:
- Total fat: 50 grams
  - Saturated fats: 8 grams

- Monounsaturated fats: 22 grams
  - Polyunsaturated fats: 9 grams
- Carbohydrates: 6 grams
  - Fiber: 1 gram
  - Carbs from sugar: 1 gram
- Protein: 17 grams

Dinner: Pesto pork chop with coleslaw

- Primary ingredients:
- 1 tablespoon of olive oil
- 2 tablespoon of salted butter
- ½ cup of shredded cabbage
- 75 grams of cooked pork chops
- 1 tablespoon of Parmesan cheese
- 1 tablespoon of basil leaves
- 1 tablespoon of mayonnaise
- Calories: 556 kcal
- Macros:
- Total fat: 52 grams
  - Saturated fats: 21 grams
  - Monounsaturated fats: 21 grams
  - Polyunsaturated fats: 6 grams
- Carbohydrates: 2 grams
  - Fiber: 1 gram
  - Carbs from sugar: 1 gram
- Protein: 21 grams

Sample Three-Day Meal Plan for Average Athletic Female Adult

Females don't typically burn as much body fat as men because of their lower base metabolic rates. This is due to the fact that the average man is going to be significantly bigger than the average woman. However, not all these principles are going to be applicable in all scenarios. This particular meal plan is going to offer a high caloric intake for an average woman. However, in this scenario, we need to take into consideration that the subject is athletic and is also likely to have higher muscle mass. This means that the subject of this meal plan is someone with a high metabolic rate to go along with a high TDEE as well. On average, a petite woman should only be consuming around 1,200–1,500 calories per day. But since this meal plan is targeting an average-sized woman who engages in regular physical activity, the average daily average is around 1,500–1,800 calories.

There is also going to be an emphasis on higher protein loads since the subject of this meal plan is someone who works out regularly and will be in need of amino acids to continually fuel her active lifestyle.

Day 1

Breakfast: Keto mac and cheese with grilled chops and buttered veggies

- ➢ Primary ingredients:
- 1 tablespoon of olive oil
- 1 tablespoon of salted butter
- ½ cup of raw cauliflower
- ½ cup of mixed vegetables
- 75 grams of grilled pork chops

- ¼ cup of cheddar cheese
- ➢ Calories: 515 kcal
- ➢ Macros:
- Total fat: 42 grams
  - Saturated fats: 17 grams
  - Monounsaturated fats: 16 grams
  - Polyunsaturated fats: 3 grams
- Carbohydrates: 11 grams
  - Fiber: 3 grams
  - Carbs from sugar: 4 grams
- Protein: 24 grams

Lunch: Pan-seared lemon butter chicken with side greens
- ➢ Primary ingredients:
- 1 tablespoon of olive oil
- 2 tablespoon salted butter
- 1 tablespoon of lemon juice
- 1 piece of chicken leg and thigh
- 50 grams of green leaf lettuce
- 50 grams of sliced cucumbers
- ➢ Calories: 536 kcal
- ➢ Macros:
- Total fat: 53 grams
  - Saturated fats: 21 grams
  - Monounsaturated fats: 22 grams
  - Polyunsaturated fats: 6 grams
- Carbohydrates: 7 grams

- Fiber: 2 grams
- Carbs from sugar: 4 grams
- Protein: 30 grams

Dinner: Low-carb Salisbury steak with creamy mushroom gravy and vegetables

- Primary ingredients:
- 1 tablespoon of olive oil
- 1 tablespoon of salted butter
- 50 grams of raw asparagus
- 15 grams of button mushrooms
- 50 ml of all-purpose cream
- 100 grams of lean ground pork
- Calories: 517 kcal
- Macros:
- Total fat: 43 grams
- Saturated fats: 9 grams
- Monounsaturated fats: 13 grams
- Polyunsaturated fats: 2 grams
- Carbohydrates: 4 grams
- Fiber: 1 gram
- Carbs from sugar: 1 gram
- Protein: 31 grams

Day 2

Breakfast: Mini mozzarella-stuffed Italian meatloaf with side greens in balsamic vinaigrette

- ➢ Primary ingredients:
- 1 slice of cheddar cheese
- 30 grams of mozzarella cheese
- 75 grams of ground pork
- 50 grams of green leaf lettuce
- 25 grams of tomatoes
- 2 tablespoon of balsamic vinaigrette
- ➢ Calories: 542 kcal
- ➢ Macros:
- Total fat: 41 grams
  - Saturated fats: 16 grams
  - Monounsaturated fats: 2 grams
  - Polyunsaturated fats 0 grams
- Carbohydrates: 12 grams
  - Fiber: 1 gram
  - Carbs from sugar: 7 grams
- Protein: 28 grams

Lunch: Low-carb cheeseburger casserole with vegetables

- ➢ Primary ingredients:
- 1 tablespoon of olive oil
- 1 ounce of cheddar cheese
- 50 milliliter of all-purpose cream
- 75 grams of lean ground pork
- ¼ cup of chopped celery

- ½ cup of sliced zucchini
- ➤ Calories: 520 kcal
- ➤ Macros:
- Total fat: 42 grams
  - Saturated fats: 9 grams
  - Monounsaturated fats: 14 grams
  - Polyunsaturated fats: 3 grams
- Carbohydrates: 5 grams
  - Fiber: 1 gram
  - Carbs from sugar: 2 grams
- Protein: 33 grams

Dinner. Pepperoni chicken pizza with side greens
- ➤ Primary ingredients:
- 1 tablespoon of olive oil
- 25 milliliters of tomato sauce
- 50 grams of mozzarella cheese
- 75 grams of cooked chicken breast
- 25 grams of sliced pepperoni
- 50 grams of green leaf lettuce
- ➤ Calories: 597 kcal
- ➤ Macros:
- Total fat: 46 grams
  - Saturated fats: 16 grams
  - Monounsaturated fats: 19 grams
  - Polyunsaturated fats: 8 grams
- Carbohydrates: 10 grams

- Fiber: 1 gram
  - Carbs from sugar: 6 grams
- Protein: 34 grams

Day 3

Breakfast: Creamy sundried tomato and crispy bacon chicken and veggies

- Primary ingredients:
- 1 tablespoon of olive oil
- 1 tablespoon of sundried tomatoes
- 1 cup of raw spinach
- 80 grams of chicken thigh
- 1 slice of bacon
- 50 milliliter of all-purpose cream
- Calories: 504 kcal
- Macros:
- Total fat: 43 grams
  - Saturated fats: 7 grams
  - Monounsaturated fats: 16 grams
  - Polyunsaturated fats: 5 grams
- Carbohydrates: 7 grams
  - Fiber: 1 gram
  - Carbs from sugar: 3 grams
- Protein: 25 grams

Lunch: Keto salad wrap with grilled chicken in VCO mayo

- ➢ Primary ingredients:
- 1 tablespoon of olive oil
- 1 tablespoon of virgin coconut oil
- ½ cup of cheddar cheese
- 80 grams of grilled chicken breast
- 50 grams of green leaf lettuce
- 50 grams of sliced cucumbers
- ➢ Calories: 640 kcal
- ➢ Macros:
- Total fat: 53 grams
  - Saturated fats: 28 grams
  - Monounsaturated fats: 18 grams
  - Polyunsaturated fats: 3 grams
- Carbohydrates: 3 grams
  - Fiber: 1 gram
  - Carbs from sugar: 1 gram
- Protein: 38 grams

Dinner: Spicy garlic chicken Parmesan wings with side greens
- ➢ Primary ingredients:
- 1 tablespoon of olive oil
- 2 tablespoon of Parmesan cheese
- 50 grams of sliced cucumbers
- 50 grams of raw carrots
- 50 grams of green leaf lettuce
- 100 grams of chicken wings
- ➢ Calories: 556 kcal

- Macros:
- Total fat: 46 grams
  - Saturated fats: 10 grams
  - Monounsaturated fats: 11 grams
  - Polyunsaturated fats: 2 grams
- Carbohydrates: 10 grams
  - Fiber: 2 grams
  - Carbs from sugar: 4 grams
- Protein: 20 grams

SUMMARY

Did you get all that? Was it a little too much? Okay. It might have been information overload for you, so as we draw this book to a close, it might be a good idea to have a little recap of the important principles and items that we have discussed here. Consider this a refresher just so you make sure that you don't forget about all the essentials.

What Is Keto?

The keto diet is a dietary program that is designed to induce a state of ketosis in the body. The term "keto" is one that stems from the word "ketones" or "ketosis." Ketosis is a metabolic state of the body in which it converts stored fat into energy to sustain daily function as opposed to relying on glucose from consumed carbohydrates. When the body is in a state of ketosis, it promotes a more efficient metabolism within the body to drive fat burn and weight loss.

Isn't Too Much Fat Bad for You?

Contrary to popular belief, the consumption of fat in itself isn't necessarily going to make you fat. This is a common misconception that a lot of people hold on to, and it's important to stress that people can get fat from proteins, carbohydrates, and other nutrients as well. The keto diet is one that actually promotes the high consumption of fat in order to induce a state of ketosis in the body. If the body has an efficient metabolic system, then it aids in the purposes of weight loss and overall fat burn. This can lead to a decreased risk of contracting obesity-related diseases and health problems.

How Do You Start Keto?

First of all, if you are looking to start the keto diet, you are going to need to do your preliminary research, and that includes reading books and other journalistic resources such as this one. Once you gain a better understanding of what the keto diet is, what it aims to achieve, and what its methodologies and principles are, then you can look into whether it's going to be a good fit for you. Take a look at your personal lifestyle and see how you will be able to tailor the keto diet around the way you live your life. It is also advisable that you consult the expertise of a licensed physician on whether the keto diet is advisable for you.

What Are Macros?

The term "macros" is something that is going to be brought up a lot in your keto journey. It's definitely a concept that you will constantly encounter because understanding your macros is key in ensuring the effectiveness of your keto program. Macros or macronutrients are the three main nutrient groups that you need to be keeping track of in your food consumption diary or journal. The three major macronutrients are fat, protein, and carbohydrates. While you are on a keto diet, you need to consume a high amount of fat, a moderate amount of protein, and a very minimal amount of carbohydrates in order to induce a ketogenic state in your body.

What Are the Three Metabolic Body Types?

In order for you to scale the keto diet to your lifestyle appropriately, you are going to want to know what kind of body type you have. There are generally only three body types, but most people are combinations of two or more body types rather than falling into a single category completely. The three body types are ectomorph, mesomorph, and endomorph.

The ectomorph is someone with a typically small and light build. They have difficulty gaining weight and building muscle. A mesomorph is someone with a more athletic build. They are still prone to weight gain, but it's easier for them to burn fat at a more efficient rate. An endomorph is someone who gains weight relatively easily, and it's harder for them to burn fat.

Can You Do Keto Even while on Vacation?

Yes. You can pretty much do keto regardless of anywhere you are in the world. One of the best things about the keto diet is just how accessible it is. You would be able to find a lot of keto-friendly food all around the world. It's all just a matter of you familiarizing yourself with the basic guidelines and principles surrounding keto and making sure that you don't compromise these principles even when you're eating outside of your comfort zone.

What's the Science behind Keto?

The science behind keto is fairly simple. It is a diet plan that is designed to maximize a person's metabolic rate in order to burn more fat throughout the day, regardless of physical activity. In order to induce a rapid rate of fat burn, the body must be engaged in a ketogenic state. The body is put into a ketogenic state when there is a lack of glucose within the human body's system, so it has to resort to the burning of stored fats in order to convert it into energy. This energy is crucial in carrying out typical body processes and sustaining human life.

Is There Such a Thing as Bad Keto?

The only ways that keto can be bad are (1) if you still adopt it in spite of the disapproval of your licensed physician and (2) if you're doing it wrong. In the latter case, it's not really a matter of keto being bad. It's more of you just practicing it mistakenly. In both cases, it doesn't mean that the keto diet is bad overall. It might just mean that it isn't a good fit for you or you're merely not executing it the way that you're supposed to.

Do You Need Supplements while on Keto?

No, you really do *not need* to be taking supplements in order for you to find success in the keto diet. However, there is no denying that using supplements healthily and responsibly can help you make the most out of your keto eating habits. If you are going to be making use of supplements, focus on taking in more nutrients that are hard to come by while you are on a keto diet. Prioritize taking electrolytes, clean protein, vitamin D, caffeine, and omega-3 fatty acids, to name a few.

What Sets Keto Apart from Other Diets?

There are many dietary philosophies and methodologies out there that are available for everyone. However, the way that the keto sets itself apart from other diets is that it doesn't really encourage bland, repetitive, and boring meals in order to promote weight loss. In fact, keto encourages a very high consumption of delicious food that can serve as great sources of fat. And with that high consumption of fat, the body produces ketones that the body converts into energy for daily activity. There are very few diets in the world (or practically none) that offer you an opportunity to eat more food in order to burn more fat. It's a unique value proposition, and that's just how it sets itself apart from other diets.

Is the Keto Diet the One for You?

Well, you never really know until you experience it for yourself. You are never going to find out just how effective the keto diet is going to be for you until you live it for yourself and see the results. It's a point that has been reiterated over and over again throughout this entire book, but it's still one that is important to stress: there is no single diet in the world that is meant for *everyone*—and that includes keto. We are all unique individuals, and we carry our own traits, preferences, tastes, and physical conditions.

The first thing you need to do is consult a licensed physician on whether the keto diet is okay for your physical makeup. And if you're cleared by your doctor, then there really isn't any harm in giving it a try, right? At the end of the day, either it works for you and you fall in love with it, or you just use it as a learning experience.

Don't Forget to Download Your Free Gift!

Scan This QR code with your smartphone or tablet and Get Your FREE GIFT NOW!

CONCLUSION

You have now essentially reached the end of this book. You are now equipped with all of the information and the guidance that you need to help you get started on your keto journey. Just keep in mind that health and fitness are always going to be a journey. It's never really about the destination because you're never really going to be done with it. You always need to be making an effort to stay fit and healthy for as long as you live. Yes, you're going to reach certain goals and milestones as you make your way through your fitness journey. But then, these goals are only going to evolve every time you reach them. So you're never really done.

And you can't be discouraged if you encounter a few hiccups along the way. You shouldn't be so quick to give up if you feel like you aren't making progress or if you're plateauing. It happens to a lot of people. As they say, nothing worth having in life is ever going to come easily. And that is why you really have to commit yourself to actually getting better at adopting a healthier and fitter lifestyle. You've already taken the first step by consulting resources and materials such as this book. That's good. It proves that you have shown initiative and that you're serious about incorporating healthier habits and practices into your own personal life.

There is no denying that it's always going to be a lot easier not to pay attention to your fitness. It can be easy to go about life just eating whatever you want and however much of it you want to eat. It's easy to focus only on your work life and relationships without paying any mind to the food that you eat or the number of minutes a day that you exercise. However, that's why a lot of people who live that "easy" life end up feeling very sick and unhealthy early on in their lives. It would be foolish to say that committing yourself to the keto diet is going to be an easy feat. It really isn't. But that's why there are books such as this one to help you make that transition to a healthier lifestyle a little bit easier.

But again, this is only the first step. Yes, it's a very big step, but it's only the first one. The acquisition of knowledge and the resolve to actually live healthier is great, but you're still going to have to go out and execute it for yourself. It's not just a matter of familiarizing yourself with the theory or telling yourself to get started. You can't just always be living in your daydreams at this point. You can't just keep on fantasizing about the healthier version of you. You need to be able to manifest all these thoughts and fantasies into reality in the form of habits and good choices. At the end of the day, you are only going to have yourself to thank for whether you become healthier or not. That's why you really need to own up to your decisions and your actions.

The road to wellness hasn't been paved to be easy or simple. It's always going to be a bumpy ride. It's always going to be an uphill climb, but you're just going to have to find a way to persevere. And if you find yourself ever feeling lost or stuck with your keto diet, don't hesitate to go back to this book for a little refresher.

Printed in Great Britain
by Amazon